SILICONE OIL IN VITREORETINAL SURGERY

SILICONE OIL IN VITREORETINAL SURGERY

Monographs in Ophthalmology

P.C. Maudgal and L. Missotten (eds.), Superficial Keratitis. 1981.
ISBN 90-6193-801-5.

P.F.J. Hoyng, Pharmacological Denervation and Glaucoma. A Clinical Trial Report with
Guanethidine and Adrenaline in One Eye Drop. 1981.
ISBN 90-6193-802-3.

N.W.H.M. Dekkers, The Cornea in Measles. 1981. ISBN 90-6193-803-1.

P. Leonard and J. Rommel, Lens Implantation − 30 years of progress. 1982.
ISBN 90-6193-804-X.

C.E. van Nouhuys, Dominant Exudative Vitreoretinopathy and Other Vascular Develop-
mental Disorders of the Peripheral Retina. 1982. ISBN 90-6193-805-8.

L. Evens (ed.), Convergent Strabismus. 1982. ISBN 90-6193-806-6.

A. Neetens, A. Löwenthal and J.J. Martin (eds.), The Visual System in Myelin Disorders.
1984. ISBN 90-6193-807-4.

H.J.M. Völker-Dieben, The Effect of Immunological and Non-Immunological Factors on
Corneal Graft Survival. 1984. ISBN 90-6193-808-2.

J.A. Oosterhuis, Ophthalmic Tumours. 1985. ISBN 90-6193-528-8.

O. van Nieuwenhuizen, Cerebral Visual Disturbance in Infantile Encephalopathy. 1987.
ISBN 0-89838-860-0.

E.A.C.M. Sanders, R.J.W. de Keizer and D.S. Zee (eds.), Eye Movement Disorders.
1987. ISBN 0-89838-874-0.

R. Živojnović, Silicone Oil in Vitreoretinal Surgery. 1987. ISBN 0-89838-879-1.

Silicone Oil in Vitreoretinal Surgery

By

R. Živojnović MD
Eye Hospital, Rotterdam, The Netherlands

1987

MARTINUS NIJHOFF/DR W. JUNK PUBLISHERS
A MEMBER OF THE KLUWER ACADEMIC PUBLISHERS GROUP
DORDRECHT / BOSTON / LANCASTER

Distributors

---

for the United States and Canada: Kluwer Academic Publishers, P.O. Box 358, Accord Station, Hingham, MA 02018-0358, USA
for the UK and Ireland: Kluwer Academic Publishers, MTP Press Limited, Falcon House, Queen Square, Lancaster LA1 1RN, UK
for all other countries: Kluwer Academic Publishers Group, Distribution Center, P.O. Box 322, 3300 AH Dordrecht, The Netherlands

Library of Congress Cataloging in Publication Data

```
Library of Congress Cataloging-in-Publication Data

Zivojnovíc, R.
    Silicone oil in vitreoretinal surgery.

    (Monographs in ophthalmology)
    Bibliography: p.
    1. Retina--Surgery.  2. Vitreous body--Surgery.
3. Silicones in surgery.  I. Title.  II. Series.
[DNLM: 1. Retina--surgery.  2. Silicone Oils.
3. Vitrectomy.  W1 MO568D / WW 270 Z82s]
RE551.Z58  1987    617.7'3059        87-7662
ISBN 0-89838-879-1 (U.S.)
```

ISBN-13: 978-94-010-7991-4   e-ISBN-13: 978-94-009-3321-7
DOI: 10.1007/978-94-009-3321-7

Copyright

Preface

With this book, Dr. Živojnović presents to the ophthalmic community the long awaited detailed report of his surgical concepts and operative techniques in the field of vitreoretinal surgery. It is fascinating to read how his concepts for the treatment of complicated retinal detachments evolved from the intraocular use of silicone oil to a combination of vitreous surgery with silicone oil tamponade. The next step was surgical treatment of the retina itself. It takes an unconventional mind to break major taboos and to state the retinotomies and retinectomies are necessary if scar tissue cannot be surgically removed and that buckling procedures are no longer necessary to treat retinal breaks.

This book discusses the use of silicone oil in vitreoretinal surgery. Silicone oil tamponade has been proven to be a major step forward in vitreoretinal surgery and the reported results speak for themselves. The reader may have the impression that silicone is thought to be indispensible for almost all cases undergoing this type of surgery but this modality is used to treat severe cases where the chances of success are greatly enhanced by using silicone oil. Dr. Živojnović remains the forerunner and great surgeon who readily admits the limitations of his techniques: 'The surgical operative treatment is only partly adequate and, unfortunately, despite the correctly performed operation, often does not lead to the desired result'.

Thus, this book not only gives a fascinating overview of the author's instrumentation, indications and surgical techniques, but it is also a stimulation to explore new avenues in the treatment of complicated retinal detachments. Thank you, Relja, for this honest account of your stimulating work!

ROBERT MACHEMER, M.D.

Contents

VIII

Introduction

Retinal surgery based on the Gonin principle of closing of the tear made great progress in the 50s due to the contributions of Custodis, Schepens, Arruga and others. Although the results were remarkably better, there was still a small number of cases that could not be treated with the new methods of indentation and bulbus shortening. Even then one recognized as the cause a process leading to practical loss of function through shrinking of the vitreous and fibrosis of the retina. Due to this process the relations between the vitreous and the retina were visibly so disturbed that they could not be influenced operatively from outside.

Introduction of the intravitreal air injection by Rosengreen was a logical attempt to approach the problem from another side. It meant an important contribution to the conventional surgery, but with complicated cases it did not bring the solution of the problem closer. Isolated publications from that time on daring instrumental interventions in the vitreous, though very plausible theoretically, found few followers because of the low technical level at that time. Following the general opinion that the problem was rooted in the vitreous, various attempts were made to find a substitute for the vitreous. For this purpose the most different biological and abiological materials were examined for their tolerance and properties.

Leaning on such experimental work on fluid silicone by Stone and Armaly, P. Cibis introduced silicone in retinal surgery in the early 60s. What was new and special in his work was that he did not use silicone as a substitute for the vitreous, but used the hydraulic power of silicone as an instrument. To make place for the injected silicone he evacuated the subretinal and intravitreal fluid and tried, under the control of a binocular ophthalmoscope, to separate the fibrotic membranes from the retina by means of the injected silicone and to press the retina against the pigment epithelium. After reattachment of the retina he left the silicone in the eye as a permanent internal tamponade. In this technique he operated several patients, inoperable according to the norms valid at that time, and achieved convincing results. Although the technique was very difficult it aroused great interest and in a very short time it was taken up by many often inexperienced and badly equipped surgeons. Technical difficulty of this technique in itself and inadequate performance of the operation under frequently bad optical control – the binocular ophthalmoscope was not in current use in Europe at that time – led to a great number of complications. All this quickly ruined the reputation of the method and it was practically abandoned in Europe in the late 60s. At the same time, Cibis' early death and administrative and legal difficulties concerning the application of silicone in the eye surgery in the USA were, on the other hand, the main reasons for abandoning this method in the USA as well.

Cibis' technique was taken up by J. Scott in Cambridge in the early 70s and further developed on a great number of patients. Following Cibis' basic principles he introduced – as crucial improvement – the vitreous scissors and other instruments for active manual surgery in the vitreous cavity. Success followed, and this method in Scott's hands offered the only hope for quite a number of desolate cases for a long time.

After D. Kasner's revolutionary clinical work in the 60s, which proved that an eye can also function without the vitreous, R. Machemer developed instrumental pars plana vitrectomy. This new and spectacular technique seemed to offer the solution for all problems in the vitreous cavity. Waiting for the expected positive results of the vitrectomy in treatment of the complicated detachment on the one hand, and a number of negative publications on the application of silicone on the other hand, were the reasons why the interest in Scott's technique, particularly in the USA, was very limited.

In the middle 70s, however, it gradually became more obvious that the expectations pinned on the vitrectomy regarding the treatment of difficult forms of retinal detachment could not be fulfilled. Although the vitrectomy was combined with the newly developed gas technique the success rate in difficult cases was less than modest. For this reason the interest in silicone and Scott's technique gradually increased.

It was the logical consequence of development that one tried to combine both techniques to further improve the results. In 1976 J. Haut in Paris injected silicone after vitrectomy for the first time and used the silicone mainly as an internal tamponade. In the last few years the application of silicone combined with the vitrectomy has spread widely in Europe, Japan and recently in the USA as well, and it has become the method of choice in treatment of difficult cases of retinal detachment in a great number of clinics.

We introduced silicone in our surgery in the beginning of 1978, after we had become convinced of the value of this technique during several visits to J. Scott in Cambridge. We operated the first few hundred cases in his original technique with the binocular ophthalmoscope and without vitrectomy. In this early

X

period pars plana vitrectomy was performed under an operation microscope only in cases with the opaque media. However, it became for us more and more obvious that the bimanual pars plana vitrectomy with its advantages was so much superior to the original Scott's method that we deserted it completely a few years ago.

Already in the beginning, operating more and more difficult cases, we found out that removal of proliferative tissue and cleaning of the retina did not suffice in some complicated cases. The retina often got incarcerated, shrunk very much or was lifted so much from the subretinal tissue that the usual vitrectomy even if combined with silicone oil failed as technique in such cases. It became clear to us that only a surgical treatment of the retina itself promised to be successful. The certainty of a permanent tamponade with silicone injection and excellent optical properties of silicone encouraged us to take this new step. New techniques of retinal surgery were consequently developed and performed as routine. Operating of the most difficult cases enabled us to have more insight in the progress and final result of the proliferative processes that we had clinically to deal with. This insight induced us further to tread more and more new paths in search of surgical success.

After more than a thousand operated cases and after a number of alterations and improvements of the technique we believe to have found a surgical concept following which we can treat most cases of complicated detachment successfully. The role of silicone in this concept, although not so domineering as in the beginning, is still decisive. Apart from the historic, revolutionary role, which – as mentioned before – enabled us to treat the retina surgically, a permanent silicone tamponade following the (performed) bimanual surgery is absolutely essential for the surgical success in cases operated in this way. Silicone has not an inhibiting influence on the further existence of a proliferative process, but beside its mechanical role as a tamponade, owing to its stabilizing effect it brings the eye into a better physiological situation and so inhibits the proliferative process indirectly. Even in cases in which the process persists and redetachment occurs, this development is much milder and slower and, due to excellent transparence of silicone, the follow-up and the treatment of these cases are much easier.

This new development in vitreoretinal surgery combined with silicone injection was accompanied by the development of new instruments which enabled realization of new ideas technically.

Due to the development of vitreoretinal surgery described before, prospects of success for many patients inoperable until a short time ago have increased enormously. It ought, though, to be remarked at once that we are fully aware of the fact that the basic problem in all cases regarded for treatment is not a surgical but a biological one. Consequently, the surgical operative treatment is only partly adequate and, unfortunately, despite the correctly performed operation, often does not lead to the desired result.

Yet, the existence of a surgical concept, the instrumental and technical progress and the surgical experience accumulated throughout the years have enabled us to operate a much larger number of difficult patients successfully than it was possible before. These facts have made me to write this book.

After having discussed the indications and the basic surgical principles of our surgery, I have described in this book the surgical techniques for various indication groups. It seemed useful to me to dedicate much space to peroperative complications. After the description of the complications I have tried to pay a lot of attention to clinical dynamics of the proliferative process, which is so important for the whole occurrence in the postoperative course.

This book does not pretend to be a textbook for advanced vitreoretinal surgery and hopes to find readers mainly with the already experienced vitreo-retinal surgeons, who encounter the problems of the proliferative process in their daily work and who are familiar with many basic notions which are not described in detail in this book.

Strictly speaking, this book has no scientific pretensions either. (Can a practical-surgical book have them at all?) Therefore the detailed bibliography given at the end of the book is not meant to be used for reference or comparison. There are many areas which, either because of lack of space or my ignorance I have not discussed sufficiently – the reader interested in them may satisfy his need by the bibliography.

Finally, I have learnt a lot in positive and negative sense from the publications on the use of silicone, which first appeared sparingly and lately have grown strong in number, and therefore they ought to be in this book.

This book is for the greatest part a history of development of a surgical conception that seems to have aroused interest lately. The conception has been developed without a previous intention and through hard clinical work. The main motivation behind the development was the permanent unsatisfaction with the achieved results.

Acknowledgements

Many individuals have contributed to the appearance of this book, to whom I wish to express my gratitude.

The book is based on my surgical experience, built up on a great number of operations and reoperations. Therefore my appreciation goes to our patients, and particularly to the Dutch patients, who have followed us on the long and uncertain road of surgical treatment unreservedly and trustfully.

My thanks go to D. Mertens, M.D., and E. Peperkamp, M.D., for the excellent cooperation and mutual support in the daily clinical work, without which the writing of this book would be inconceivable, as well as for their conscientious revising of the manuscript. My particular thanks go to D. Mertens for the assistance with compiling of the bibliography.

I would like to thank Mr. Vijfvinkel and his collaborators for the long-standing cooperation in the development of new instruments and for the technical description of the instruments in this book.

I also thank the photography department, particularly B. Smit and D. de Bruin for their readiness and professional work in the past years and for their contribution in this book.

My thanks go to Prof.Dr. V.P. Gabel for his willing assistance in writing the chapter on properties of silicone.

Mrs. D. Verhoeven deserves my particular thanks for the technical assistance in preparation of the manuscript.

I thank Mr. Tiets who has designed drawings in this book.

I would also like to thank Prof.Dr. P. Kroll for stimulating discussions concerning the decision to write this book.

A great part of this book has come into being in the operating theatre, therefore I would like to express my thanks and appreciation for the good cooperation to G. Griese and all collaborators in the theatre.

Last but not least I would like to thank my wife Vesna. She deserves this appreciation not only for accepting the difficulties of my professional life – the appearance of this book will change little in it – but much more for the translation of the manuscript and her constructive criticism.

1. Indications

Use of silicone oil in vitreoretinal surgery is indicated mainly in the pathological changes generated by a proliferative process. The most frequent proliferative changes in the treatment of which the use of silicone oil is indicated are:

1. proliferative vitreoretinopathy (PVR) generated spontaneously after a long existing retinal detachment or after an unsuccessful detachment surgery;
2. retinal detachment with PVR after perforating injuries;
3. spontaneous or secondary developed giant tears of the retina with or without detachment; and
4. traction detachment in the diabetic retinopathy.

In addition to these four large indication groups, which form the greatest part of the cases, this technique is indicated in the rare secondary traction detachments following inflammatory process as well as in traction detachments with retinopathy of prematurity (ROP). A relative indication are the detachment cases with a hole in posterior pole and mobile retina, which may also be treated in various other techniques and without silicone.

The above-given introduction to various indication groups suggests simplicity and clearness in establishing a diagnosis and classifying of pathological changes, which is by no means so in practice. The proliferative process in the most difficult forms of retinal detachment has been recognized clinically for years. It consists of cell proliferations and contraction of newly grown membranes, and in the past had various names, e.g. massive vitreal retraction (MVR), massive preretinal retraction (MPR) or massive periretinal proliferation (MPP). The latest name, proliferative vitreoretinopathy (PVR) is a fairly adequate description, although it suggests that the process involves only the retina and the vitreous, which is by no means true in a number of situations. While the terminological discussion seems to be finished with a fair result for the time being, it is completely different with the classification of various phases and grades of difficulty of the clinical process. The need for such a classification was to be seen already with the first attempt at a surgical treatment. In the discussion on indications and surgical results the diagnosis alone was not sufficient, and a closer description of cases and their classification proved necessary. A great number of attempts from the past to describe and classify various phases of the proliferative process only shows the imperfection of each attempt and, at the same time, the difficulty of the task.

Even the latest classification of the Retina Society is, unfortunately, not much more than an honourable attempt to fulfill this difficult task.

An optimal and usable classification should not only take into account the fundus picture of the posterior retina, but should also include the changes of the peripheral retina and the vitreous base. Further, the number, size and location of the retinal tears are of great importance for the course of the operation and for the prognosis. Even if one could describe and classify the above mentioned changes and their mutual relationships, it would be only a momentary and static picture of the pathological situation. For further judgement the duration of the process and stages of development are very important, which can only partly be read from the fundus picture. Further, even if the mobility of the retina and the vitreous can be evaluated to some extent by a preoperative examination, the preoperative judgement on the firmness of adhesion between membranes and the retina is impossible. This will be discovered, as so many other things, only during the operation. Exactly the same holds for the existence of subretinal proliferations, which are very often detected only during the operation. The pre-history and etiology of a single case are decisive for the course of the proliferative process. This concerns in particular the trauma cases that very often look much more harmless than they really are and should, probably, best be classified separately.

Referring to all these factors important for the classification we only want to point out difficulties one meets with when talking about the precise indications for application of the silicone oil.

It is evident that the silicone as foreign substance may be used only in otherwise inoperable cases. Although the number of complications has been considerably reduced through the improved technique, the first complication of the silicone injection is the silicone itself which is in the eye and has to be removed as soon as possible. Even without taking into account possible complications, the removal of the silicone already means a second operation for the patient. Therefore, in our opinion, not all cases in the before-named indication groups may promptly be treated with the silicone, vitrectomy, etc., but in some of them an attempt at conventional surgery is justified. On the other hand we believe that when in such cases the conventional surgery (encircling band, buckle, etc.) has not been successful and the proliferative process is progressing, one has to try the silicone and vitrectomy immediately so as to offer the patient the greatest opportunity for success.

2

It seems necessary to us, just because there is no usable classification, to explain more thoroughly the indications for the use of silicone in various indication groups.

PVR after idiopathic retinal detachment

From time to time we come across cases of longer existing retinal detachments which have not been operated for various reasons, and which besides the open hole, i.e. the rhegmatogenous element, also display signs of a beginning or advanced PVR. The detachment is mostly subtotal or total, with a star fold, curled tear edges and other symptoms of a PVR. As we know even from the time when we did not have in our arsenal such powerful means as silicone and vitrectomy, these cases, treated with conventional surgery, were not all lost. Therefore we believe that an attempt at a conventional operation is worth trying. A gentle encircling element with a radial buckle, drainage and possibly salt solution or gas-air mixture injection can be successful in approximately 50% of these cases. Some of these successfully operated cases later develop a macula pucker, which, again, can be operated successfully in a quiet phase after a few months. In cases where detachment still exists after the conventional surgery and the proliferative process is progressing, a combined operation with vitrectomy and silicone oil is, in our opinion, indicated immediately. A number of these cases may also be successfully operated with vitrectomy and gas mixture. There will probably always remain a grey indication zone where both surgery techniques overlap and where, in some cases, silicone oil is used unnecessarily. What seems to us even more important is the fact that if a case has already been unsuccessfully operated with vitrectomy and gas-air mixture, it has a worse anatomical and much worse functional prognosis with a following silicone operation.

The use of silicone oil as the first operation should occur exceptionally in one-eyed patients as well as in very old patients. We would, namely, prefer not to burden both groups with the prospect of several operations, at the same time we would like to achieve in them good functional results as soon as possible. Vitrectomy with the use of silicone oil in the first operation offers these patients just the best opportunity for it. The disadvantage that afterwards there is silicone oil in the eye, which necessitates a second operation at a later time, has to be put up with in this group of patients.

The second group of patients are the cases with retinal detachment and PVR, who have been conventionally operated without success one or more times. In these patients the proliferative process is in full progress, the defects, i.e. the rhegmatogenous element, plays no or just a subordinate role, and in these patients the use of silicone is indicated almost without exception.

Retinal detachments with and without PVR developed after a perforating trauma

The mechanism of the development of a retinal detachment after a perforating injury is manifold and corresponding to different pathoanatomic situations. Therefore, it seems important to us, before discussing the use of silicone oil in different situations, to examine the components of this mechanism.

In the severe perforating trauma, mostly in the lacerating injuries with the expressed lens, iris and vitreous, the retinal detachment is due to the mechanical traction directly at the injury. After the injury the retina is either incarcerated in the perforation wound or, more frequently, connected to the wound through the incarcerated vitreous. The created situation becomes worse through the contraction caused by the scarring process. The scarring process is a normal reparative activity as the answer of the organism to the perforating trauma. In smaller injuries this process can end without great damage or with a local traction without going into a proliferative and aggressive process. In the severe perforating injuries, particularly in those with directly developed retinal detachment, there is a great probability of development of the proliferative process together with, or secondary to, the scarring process. Comprehension of the above mentioned phenomenon and clinical experience give us the possibility to judge the given situation and to decide whether in the single case the conventional technique or the silicone oil should be used. Following the diagnostics of the pathoanatomical process, we would like to discuss each group concerning the treatment. In the patients who have a retinal detachment combined with a severe trauma and loss of substance (lens, vitreous, iris), the use of silicone oil in the first operation is certainly justified. The development of the proliferative process in such cases is nearly unavoidable and the waiting for it or the application of the conventional technique only means repeated surgery in a more difficult situation.

The eyes that have come through a perforating injury without retinal detachment can sometimes still develop one after a few weeks or months. Retinal detachment develops during the scarring process through the direct traction on the surroundings or, very often through the traction of the vitreous on the opposite peripheral retina. This has nothing to do with a proliferative process but with the mechanical traction generated by the contraction of the scar, which is an adequate reparative process. In such a situation it is possible to succeed with conventional surgery.

In case of failure in such cases a proliferative process often starts developing. In that case one should not hesitate to use silicone oil and vitrectomy in the following operation.

A very serious group of patients are the cases which most probably got the detachment mechanically with the injury, but which were not directly recognized for objective or subjective reasons. These cases come for treatment several weeks or months after the injury. The retina is mostly completely organized and often incorporated in the perforation scars. There is no doubt that only a very radical operation with silicone oil injection can offer these eyes a small and modest chance of success.

Giant tears

It is not our intention to write here on the pathogenesis and diagnostics of giant tears, but for the reason of clearness we want to emphasize that neither big ora tears nor very big equatorial tears belong to this indication group. Both have a completely different mechanism of development and should be treated with conventional methods. Development of a giant tear is a dramatic process with typical symptoms, and always leads to a total detachment and PVR. The prodromes of development of tears with the subsequent detachment can be understood, in our view, as an early stage of the proliferative process of the PVR. Therefore not only the size of the tear but also the size of detachment, the mobility of the retina and the presence of other symptoms of the PVR are decisive for the prognosis and the choice of the surgical method. All enumerated symptoms of this pathological process deteriorate increasingly with time, sometimes even with hours. Therefore the time of generation of the process is also of great relevance.

Seriousness of the situation and the prognosis with giant tears regarding the development of the PVR and the relatively poor results with other methods (a great number of redetachments) reinforced our opinion that most giant tears should be treated with vitrectomy and silicone oil injection. A very limited number of giant tears that come to treatment in a very early stage can be treated with gas-air mixture injection and vitrectomy. Especially tears in upper part of the retina without retinal detachment and with a short case history are suitable for such treatment.

Diabetic traction detachment

Pars plana vitrectomy proved successful as the surgical method just in the treatment of diabetic retinopathy and nowadays it is certain that a major part of the cases can be operated successfully in this way. The proliferative process in the diabetic retinopathy has a different nature from PVR, and the removal of vitreous and fibrotic tissue as well as release of mechanical traction leads to success in many cases. There is still a rather large group of cases which are considered to be difficult to operate. These are the cases with long existing total or subtotal retinal detachment, very strong fibrovascular membranes prone to bleeding and frequently with a rhegmatogenous element too. In the last year this group of patients was often, just because of numerous postoperative complications after vitrectomy, such as secondary glaucoma and phthisis, excluded from treatment and regarded as inoperable. Through absence of postoperative hypotony and bleeding after a silicone oil injection, and perhaps through other still hypothetic factors, the number of postoperative complications after a silicone oil injection is surprisingly small. In these desolate cases good anatomical results are achieved with vitrectomy combined with retinal surgery and silicone oil injection.

A second indication for the use of silicone oil in diabetics is in the patients with strong inclination to postoperative bleeding. In these patients retinal detachment is not prominent, it even does not exist at all, but silicone oil is used to stabilize the eye. Through the silicone oil injection, postoperative hypotony and secondary haemorrhage are avoided and the possibility is created to treat the retina postoperatively with laser photocoagulation. This is an arbitrary indication which is particularly suitable in psychically strained or one-eyed patients for whom it is psychically difficult to cope with secondary hemorrhage after operation.

The above-named and described indications are based on our clinical experience from the time before we used silicone oil and on the basis of our experience with more than a thousand cases operated with silicone oil in the last 8 years. Although we are convinced that for the time being no better results in these difficult cases can be achieved with any other technique, we believe that the decision to use silicone oil has to be examined in every single case again. Silicone oil may cause various complications after some time and it should best be removed as soon as possible. However, silicone oil has no direct influence on the proliferative process, which again in many cases progresses and causes the changes that, provisionally, make the removal of silicone oil impossible. The solution is then to operate further, which means a new strain for the patient and a new uncertainty concerning the final result.

In this complicated and difficult situation, the patient and the surgeon, it seems to us very useful to define a little more closely the prospects of the success of surgery. Although all statistic results, particularly in patients so hard to compare, are certainly of a very limited value, we would like to give the probability of success for each main indication group in Table 1. This table has been put together on account of the results of the last 2 years, when the technique was already stabilized and practically not changed. Of course, the desirable operation to remove silicone oil has to be added to every successfully operated case.

6

The pathoanatomic point of view, which we have discussed by now, is, of course, fundamental, but not the only one decisive for the indication for an operation. The pathoanatomic basis of an indication shows that an operation is possible and not useless; whether it should be performed is another question. Just in this – in every aspect – difficult pathology with complicated treatment techniques, uncertain final results and a long way to a possible success, it seems very important to us to concern ourselves also with ethic and practical-clinical points of view of this problem.

The one-eyed patients in whom a right pathoanatomic indication has been made are the smallest problem here; if they still have positive light perception in the last eye, they have to be operated, as otherwise they will become blind. The functional monoculi in whom the relevant eye used to be the better one are an intermediary group, but the problem gets truly complicated if the other eye has a good function.

The operating of the so-called second eye will always depend on the opinion of the surgeon, the motivation of the patient and numerous other conditions. As it is, for this reason, very difficult to give rules, it seems useful to us to enlighten more closely a few aspects important for making the decision. The general criteria valid for the operation of the second eye such as the condition of the good eye (possible belonging to one of the risk groups like myopia, congenital cataract, etc.), further age and life expectation of the patient, internal and psychic condition, must also, naturally, be taken into account.

The most important question after that is what is the use for the patient of the expected anatomic success.

The functional success is marked more by regained visual field than by the central vision, which mostly turns out very modest. The possible security to have one, even if poor eye in reserve for future is highly estimated by many patients. Absence of possible complications (secondary glaucoma, phthisis), which sometimes may appear even without surgery (although not to be proved in a single case), could also be an advantage of a successful operation.

The disadvantages of the operation would be the usual risk, postoperative discomfort and the development of complications. The difficulties are not

Table 1. Probability of success for various indication groups – probability of a second operation in parentheses.

Indication group	
PVR after idiopathic retinal detachment	90–95% (30–40%)
PVR after perforating trauma	70–75% (50–60%)
Giant tears with and without PVR	90–95% (30–40%)
Diabetic traction detachment	80–90% (20–30%)

great and the number of complications has become significantly lower with the new development of the technique.

The greatest disadvantage of the whole treatment is the uncertainty concerning the number of necessary operations and the final success. The fact that the surgical treatment is not totally adequate for the solution of the problem and that the process progresses in spite of initially good results of the operation and leads to a redetachment, is perhaps still plausible to a diabetic but very incomprehensible to any other patient. His motivation, still very strong before the first silicone operation, disappears increasingly with every new half-successful operation and his inclination to break off the treatment before the end grows. To prevent this and to convince the patient further into justification of a treatment in spite of uncertain final results, is the difficult task of the surgeon.

Thereby we have come to the key problem of the surgical treatment of proliferative processes altogether. Repeated surgery in irregular periods and regular follow-up between the operations represent a great problem for the patients in every respect. Therefore, especially in the patients with the good second eye a strong temptation appears in the course of time to break off the treatment and so to annihilate the achieved result.

It is obvious from the hitherto stated that a talk with the patient before the operation is of decisive importance. In this talk, not only positive prospects on the basis of pathoanatomic situation, but also all other aspects have to be discussed in detail.

The existing possibility of several operations and the removal of silicone oil have to be mentioned. At the same time it should be explained that the initially good results can often be permanently secured only with several operations and that breaking off of the treatment would most probably annihilate the result. Finally, the patient should also hear what he has always wanted to know but has not dared to ask, what will happen with the eye if the operation does not succeed. He should hear that such eyes usually do not cause great subjective troubles (the trauma eyes sometimes excluded) and seldom become atrophic.

One should not spare either pains or time to have such a talk with the patient before the operation. With this talk, not only necessary information is given to the patient but also a basis of confidence is created for the often very long way to be covered together to the desired success.

Many misunderstandings and disappointments, and trying the other clinic, which was frequently to be seen in long treated patients, could have been avoided by a good talk before the first operation.

2. Surgical principles

The surgical principles that we want to explain are based on a surgical concept that we have developed in the last years. This concept was not a product of a momentary inspiration, which is easy to understand, but has been built up gradually and not always in a straight line. The development of this concept is for the greatest part due to the use of silicone oil. Although nowadays silicone oil plays a much smaller part than it did in the beginning, many new steps in the development of this surgery were only imaginable and possible because one was aware of the possibility and the certainty of an inner tamponade after the silicone oil injection.

The aggressivity and persistence of the proliferative processes we had to treat showed us that conventional surgical methods failed in most cases. It appeared repeatedly that the learned and existing surgical principles in the ophthalmic surgery presented a burden rather than a help. The cautious, defensive surgery was too frequently without effect, radical interventions often done in desperate and hopeless situations sometimes, surprisingly, brought the desired success. Gradually we have become convinced that in these difficult cases, attacked by the aggressive proliferative process, only correspondingly radical and aggressive surgery can succeed. However, as always, this concept also has its disadvantage caused by the process itself. It is, namely, certain that each intervention and each treatment during the operation can provoke and propagate the process. This danger is almost unavoidable and can only be decreased by as atraumatic surgery as possible. Balancing between the necessary surgical aggressivity and the yearning to keep the surgical trauma within limits is a difficult task. Fulfillment of this task will strongly influence the final success of the surgery.

Before we start explaining in particular principles serving as the basis of the concept, we would like briefly to pay our attention to the Scott's method. Although the original Scott's technique has been partly abandoned also by Scott himself, this technique is the basis and the beginning of the whole progress recorded in the vitreoretinal surgery in the last years.

The original Scott's technique is always identified with the binocular ophthalmoscope. It is true that the binocular ophthalmoscope was used there to observe the progress of surgery. The same, however, can be done with the microscope. The binocular ophthalmoscope has the advantage of a larger visual field and better mobility at observation of the progress. On the other hand the working in the upright picture and better visibility are the great advantages of the microscope. It is fundamental in Scott's technique, though, that silicone oil is used as the instrument to dissect membranes from the retina and to unfold the retina.

The somewhat too simple Cibis' idea to start the silicone oil injection in front of the disc and to inject silicone oil between the retina and membranes appeared too difficult and complicated in many cases. Besides, through its lighter specific gravity silicone oil tended to drift upward in the aqueous environment and transform into many little bubbles, which seriously impeded visibility (Figs. 1 and 2). J. Scott injected silicone oil immediately behind the lens and that was his first great contribution to improvement of the silicone oil technique. After the drainage of the intravitreal space to create place for silicone oil, silicone oil is injected behind the lens, if possible immediately behind the anterior vitreous. By further injecting, the silicone oil bubble was pushed backwards, broke the fibrotic structures and, if existing, the posterior vitreous membrane and came in the posterior pole in contact with the retina (Figs. 3 and 4). Once in contact with the retina, the further expansion power brought the silicone oil under the vitreous or fibrotic membranes and separated these from the retina.

The situation was more difficult when the retina was partly or completely covered with epiretinal membranes. As the retina is longer and more elastic than the membranes lying upon it, in a favourable case the membranes broke up and the retina straightened and became attached. With very adherent membranes the power of silicone oil expansion, difficult to control, could tear the retina. To avoid this, J. Scott introduced intraocular instruments in this technique, which represented a further and decisive improvement. The membranes were lifted from the retina surface with the dissection needle and the fibrotic structures were cut with the vitreous scissors, and in this way the space was created for further expansion of the silicone oil. All this was going on simultaneously with the further removal of intravitreal and subretinal fluid. The favourable development of the process was always endangered by pressure on existing retinal tears, which are connected to the proliferative membranes in different ways, e.g. with a tear flap. At the expansion of the silicone oil bubble the membranes and the retina are separated by tension.

If there were existing tears in this area or newly developed tears caused by traction of silicone oil expansion, the silicone oil came under the retina. That meant a catastrophe in two aspects and frequently the end of the operation.

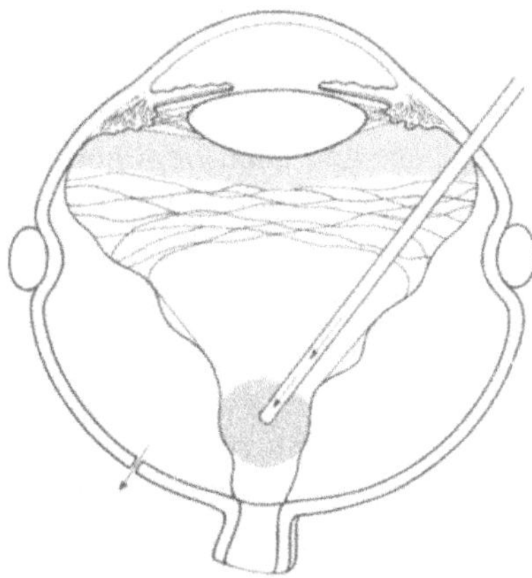

Figure 1. Use of silicone as an instrument – technique after P. Cibis.

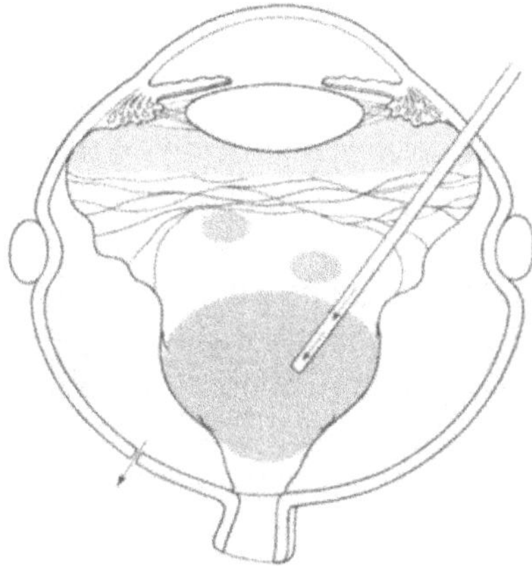

Figure 2. Use of silicone as an instrument – technique after P. Cibis.

First, in the situation when the silicone oil is both in the intravitreal and subretinal space, its expansive power cannot be used anymore, and with further injecting more and more silicone oil would come behind the retina. Second, the silicone oil was very difficult to remove from behind the retina and therefore the closing of the hole was often impossible. For this reason the closing of the tear before the silicone oil injection was an absolute precondition which was not always so easy to achieve.

If the operation took a favourable turn, which happened often enough, at the end of the operation there was one single silicone bubble posterior in a good contact with the retina, separated from the lens by anterior vitreous or membrane layer. However, in the farthest retina periphery and to the ciliary body a peripheral retinal detachment was frequently to be seen because the expansion power of the silicone oil did not reach this zone. This retinal detachment was connected to and held upright by circular fibrotic structures connected to the vitreous base and ciliary epithelium. For the further post-opertive course these peripheral proliferations proved a time bomb, which spontaneously or with each new intervention (e.g. cataract surgery) turned the original success to failure through reproliferation and subsequent traction.

The original Scott's technique was only applicable in fairly clear media and in cases in which no massive fibrotic structures or foreign bodies had to be removed from the eye.

The peroperative complications, such as a retinal tear with silicone oil behind the retina, a chorioidal or retinal bleeding, were not so frequent, but once developed they were difficult to treat without controlled eye pressure, unimanually and with frequently bad fundus view, and the eye had to be abandoned. This technique was difficult but fascinating, it demanded from the surgeon not only perfect skill but also control and good interpretation of the whole procedure. Therefore, every mistake and negligence of every misin-terpretation was immediately punished.

Not taking into account technical difficulty of this technique, which made the success of the surgery highly dependable on the individual qualities of a single surgeon, the limitations it implied became incompatible with the further development and subsequent demands in the surgery.

For these reasons, to improve in this way the imperfection of the technique in various phases of the operation, Scott also introduced vitrectomy in this technique. He performed vitrectomy after silicone oil injection using the silicone oil still as an instrument, and vitrectomy served to remove the vitreous and various other structures outside the silicone bubble.

For the same reasons we have abandoned this technique after having it used intensely for a few years. Bimanual pars plana vitrectomy enables us to free the retina from the proliferative tissue in a much better, more secure and more perfect way. The infusion line from the beginning of the operation and the consequent eye pressure control give us not only the possibility of comfortable surgery under good optical control but also the possibility of treatment of all peroperative complications, which are anything but rare in this excessive surgery. The high level of security offered by this technical system enables us to remove fibrotic structures, scar tissues and foreign bodies. The last and also the most important argument is that the bimanual pars plana vitrectomy with the comfortable security of the whole system encouraged us to treat such difficult cases as were certainly not treatable with the original Scott's method. In this new concept, silicone oil is hardly at all used as an instrument but much more as an inner tamponade and as a stabilizer of the situation reached by vitrectomy.

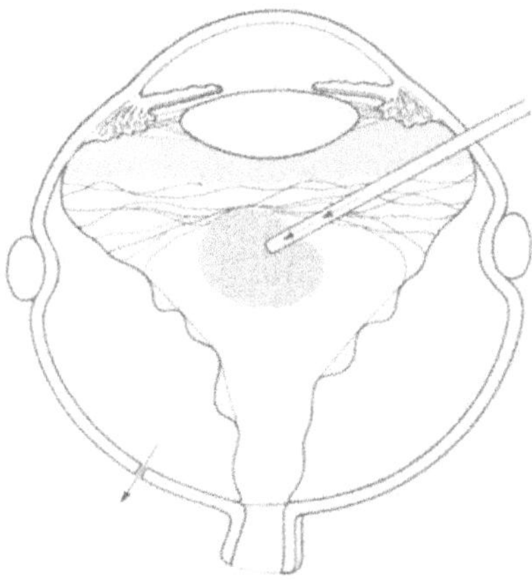

Figure 3. Use of silicone as an instrument – technique after J. Scott.

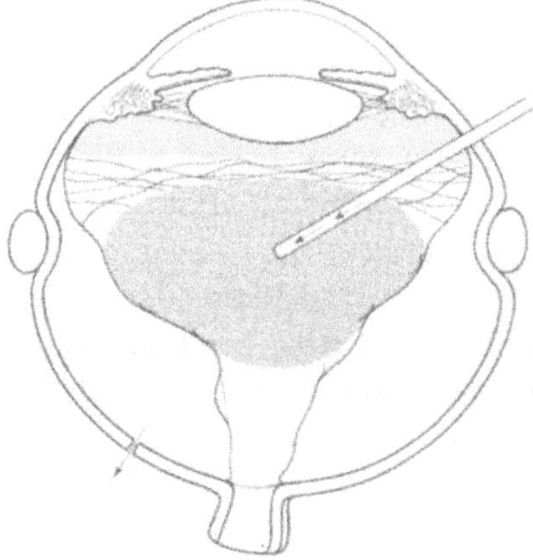

Figure 4. Use of silicone as an instrument – technique after J. Scott.

Silicone oil as an active instrument is still used only for reposition of the mobilized retina. The retina is mobile at the end of the operation, unfolded and free from the fibrotic tissue and as such it should be attached yet with the silicone injection. In this phase silicone oil and its expansion power is used as an instrument to reattach the retina. With the simultaneous endodrainage the retina is gently pressed against the pigment epithelium under the control of the microscope and bimanual help of the instruments.

Silicone oil as a passive instrument is mostly used at reoperations when silicone oil was already injected at the first operation. The advantage of the silicone oil in the eye is its excellent transparency securing good view during the surgery. Further, silicone oil, through its surface tension and viscosity holds the retina in the position, which makes the removal of epiretinal membranes from the retina surface significantly easier. Simultaneously, the lifted membranes have become much better visible through the different refractive index of silicone oil. The regular intraocular pressure during surgery, very important for the constant conditions, is secured by the adjustable infusion of silicone oil.

Once in the eye silicone oil serves as a permanent inner tamponade and a stabilizer of the existing conditions. The two roles cannot be separated and ought to be discussed together.

The effect of the inner silicone oil tamponade is too frequently understood as a purely mechanical effect. This view is, in our opinion, too simple and does not correspond to the facts. The mechanical power of the silicone oil tamponade corresponds only to the driving force and the mass of the silicone oil bubble and is not comparable to e.g. the mechanical force of a fixed episcleral buckle. Also the contact of the silicone oil bubble with the retina is only indirect as there is always a layer of fluid between the two and is not comparable to the ideal contact of an air or gas bubble with the retina. One should also remember that during the surgery the complete filling of the eye with silicone oil is often not possible for various reasons (e.g. existence of chorioidal swelling, failure of complete fluid evacuation). As silicone oil after the injection has no expansion power, after receding of swelling or absorption of the fluid there is in such cases always an additional space not filled with silicone oil. Finally it can be remarked that also this gentle and moderate mechanical effect is not always the same and in the same place through the change of the position of the head.

If one takes these facts into consideration, it becomes clear that the positive effect of the silicone oil tamponade is only to be found in the interaction with other factors.

The most important of these factors is the state of the retina. A mobile, not contracted retina, free of every vertical and tangential traction tends to attach itself and does not need much mechanical pressure to stay attached. This tendency is supported by the good function of the pigment epithelium pump, which has a positive role as the second factor. It is well known that the fluid circulation in the eye has a negative influence on the attachment of the retina. In eyes filled with silicone oil the amount of fluid and so also the circulation outside the silicone oil bubble is reduced to a minimum. The postoperative attachment of the retina is the result of the presence of positive factors as mechanical tamponade, the mobile retina, good function of the pigment epithelium pump and absence of negative factors as any kind of traction and fluid circulation. This result is corroborated by the development of retinopexy scars on the long term supported and assured by the permanent silicone oil tamponade. The role of the retinal holes will be discussed at length later on,

14

but it may be said immediately that they do not take an important part in the whole procedure. Their role can become important only in combination with other factors such as newly existing traction. The complete reattachment of the retina achieved through vitrectomy and the silicone oil injection can be secured for a shorter or longer time owing to the joint effect of the inner silicone oil tamponade and other mentioned factors.

Preservation of good surgical results for a longer period is completely dependent on development of proliferative processes in the first postoperative weeks. Silicone oil in the eye can, as already mentioned, not directly influence the biologic process of proliferation, but it can with its presence in the eye eliminate or inhibit other factors which stimulate the proliferative process.

We think here of postoperative hypotony with all its consequences, postoperative bleeding, further exudation and inflammatory reaction occurring after extensive surgery. When present in the eye in the optimum quantity, silicone oil has a positive stabilizing effect. Even when the proliferative process is in progress, this development – under silicone oil – is slower, less dramatic and owing to its excellent optic quality completely controllable.

The stabilizing effect of silicone oil is clinically provable, occurs immediately after surgery and cannot be separated in time from the mechanical effect of the inner tamponade. To achieve both, the eye has to be optimally filled with silicone oil. The optimum filling is dependent on many factors in the given situation and not measurable. There are, though, a few rules that can be followed to achieve the optimum filling: vitrectomy or removal of everything that one has intended to remove has to be performed as completely as possible. Evacuation of intraocular and subretinal fluid has also to be as complete as possible. The silicone oil bubble has to fill the whole posterior segment and to stay behind the diaphragm, the anterior chamber has to be deep and free from silicone oil, the eye pressure has to be normal at the end of the surgery.

As we have already indicated, the role of retinal defects is, in this surgical concept, of secondary importance. This perhaps surprising statement can be understood better if one remembers the mechanism of the development of retinal detachment and its treatment with the conventional surgery. For the development of retinal detachment three factors are generally essential: traction on the retina, the hole and the circulation of fluid (the sequence may be different). The retinal detachment is cured most rapidly when the hole is completely closed with an external buckle after evacuation of the subretinal fluid. But closing of the hole during the surgery is not absolutely necessary for the cure. It is sufficient if the buckle is put on the right place under the hole. In this way the vitreous traction is eliminated and the local fluid circulation is decreased through changed relations between the retina and the vitreous. Because of decreased inflow of the fluid the absorptive capacity of the pigment epithelium pump suffices to absorb the subretinal fluid. The distance between the buckle and the retina is reduced and finally the hole is completely closed. The whole will function in the described way only if the retina is completely mobile. In the whole process the retina has no active role, but must not offer a passive resistance either. If the retina is contracted and immobile, the contact between the buckle and the retina will not take place, the hole will remain open and the detachment will persist.

The same mechanism is valid for the situation developed after vitrectomy and silicone oil injection. Only the relations are changed: the vitreous-retina traction is completely eliminated, the circulation of fluid is strongly decreased through the silicone oil injection and can be neglected, the retinal hole exists but the mobile retina is gently reattached by the silicone bubble. In the described situation there are further no mechanical factors that may cause a rhegmatogenous detachment. The retinal hole can be immediately closed with endolasercoagulation or will be closed with the cryopexy after development of chorioretinal scars a week after the surgery. Absence of rhegmatogenous detachment will certainly not be due to retinopexy and closing of the holes.

The redetachment developed a few days or weeks after surgery, which is unfortunately seen too frequently, has its origin in reproliferation of the new or pre-existing proliferative membranes. The retinal holes that are often to be seen after reoccurrence of detachment are secondary developed by the traction. An indenting operation performed in combination with vitrectomy and silicone oil injection will change nothing in this process. As it does not treat the cause but the consequence it will hardly prevent the development of detachment but at best perhaps only detain it.

For these reasons there is in our surgical concept practically no more place for indenting surgery. A cerclage is still used as routine only to present better the peripheral retina during vitrectomy. The role of vitrectomy in this concept has become more and more important with the development in the last years. Under the term of vitrectomy is not only meant the removal of the vitreous but all intraocular structures that should be removed during the operation. It concerns newly developed epiretinal membranes and fibrotic tissue developed after former operations and trauma. The purpose of vitrectomy or rather of the removal of vitreous and fibrotic structures is first the elimination of traction and the mobilization of the retina. The retina, though, can become completely mobile only when it has been cleaned of all epiretinal membranes. The cleaning of the retina is a very important phase of the operation and has to be performed with the necessary perfection and as atraumatically as possible. Difficulties are presented by unripe membranes, which are very difficult to recognize.

A further but very important role of vitrectomy is the removal of all tissue that can potentially become a scaffolding for possible proliferations in the future. The removal of the potential scaffolding is not the same as the elimina-

16

tion of traction. Particularly in the fresh cases with PVR the vitreous on the vitrous base need not yet be contracted under circumstances and in this case the traction on the retina will not be visible. If one does not remove the peripheral vitreous misled by relatively good appearance of the retinal periphery, one will be punished later with the peripheral contraction and redetachment. It will not be different with the other peripheral tissue.

The experience has shown us that the proliferative process under the silicone oil often proceeds and does not confine itself to the posterior part of the eye. In this progress every tissue that is in the way is used as a scaffolding. In the course of years we have transferred the focal point of our interest more and more to the periphery, which does not imply that the posterior pole was neglected. In the cases where we first were satisfied with the attached retina posterior to the buckle, we had to observe after some time that the retina was redetached through peripheral traction. The development of the redetachment through the peripheral traction in the late postoperative phase induced us to pay more and more attention to the vitreous base. The proliferation in the area of the vitreous base with the subsequent traction has its effect not only upon the central retina but also on the ciliary body. The central detachment developed first from this process is in difficult cases later followed by the ciliary body atrophy and hypotony. Particularly difficult forms of this process are seen in the perforative injuries, where the proliferation progresses directly from the perforation scar. The proliferative process in difficult cases can only temporarily be influenced by palliative measures such as indenting operation combined with cryopexy. With a radical vitrectomy in the area of the vitreous base, in which not only the vitreous but also all newly developed structures and lens remnants are removed, the existing traction is eliminated and the scaffolding for future traction removed. At the same time the function of the ciliary body is secured.

At this point the question arises what is the role of the lens in the whole concept. The role of the lens has continuously changed in this surgery. In the beginning, in the original Scott's technique the lens was regarded as protection against penetrating of silicone oil into the anterior segment. The lens, preferably with some vitreous behind it, was tried to be preserved. Although in most treated eyes the lens was not in direct contact with silicone oil, the majority of patients developed cataract within a year. That meant reduction of the function and disappointment for the patient. For many patients with the good second eye that frequently meant the point of breaking off the treatment and cancelling further surgery. For the others that meant a new operation, which was often followed by revival of the proliferative process and redetachment.

With the increased application of vitrectomy the lens was more difficult to protect, silicone oil came more frequently beside the lens into the anterior chamber and the cataract occurred earlier than before. At that time one already had the feeling that the lens was sometimes more disturbing than useful, but there was always fear of silicone oil in the anterior chamber and subsequent difficulties with the cornea and it warned us against extraction of the clear lens. The introduction of the peripheral iridectomy at 6 o'clock, by which silicone oil remains in the posterior part of the eye, has made the fears superfluous for the greatest part. For some time now we have removed the lens at the first silicone oil operation and we believe that advantages of a lens extraction surpass disadvantages. If possible the lens is removed through the pars plana. For the already mentioned reasons a lot of attention is also paid to the removal of the zonula fibres and the lens remnants. The removal of the clear lens saves the patient a second operation, which often represents the cause of new complications. It secures a constant and good fundus view after the surgery, which is of great importance for the control of the postoperative process.

In the original Scott's technique the drainage of subretinal fluid occurred from outside through a sclerotomy, mostly parallel to the injection of silicone oil. Besides all the known risks such as chorioidal hemorrhage, uncontrollable intraocular pressure, etc., the difficulty was also that the process could be observed from one side only, either from inside or from outside, which made the control of the drainage difficult. Consequently, at the development of complications the corresponding measure could not be applied in time.

In the new surgical concept, in which the whole surgical procedure takes place inside the eye, it is quite natural that the subretinal fluid is evacuated from inside and under the control through the microscope. In this way the whole process is well controllable and the peroperative complications are extremely rare. As with any other treatment, there are also certain disadvantages. At the evacuation of the subretinal fluid it is necessary, as well known, to introduce the instrument under the retina. As long as it is done through the already existing retinal defects, and the pigment epithelium is not damaged, it will pass unnoticed and without consequences. But if this is not possible, the only possibility to perform the evacuation of the subretinal fluid inside the eye is to make an iatrogenic retinal hole, i.e. a retinotomy. Although a small retinotomy passes in most cases without complications, sometimes there are complications in the postoperative course that, with more caution, can be avoided. Great importance has to be given to the position of retinotomy. The surrounding retina should be completely free of epiretinal membranes. Manipulating of instruments should also occur very carefully, every unnecessary damage of the chorioidea or the retina can be the cause of future reproliferation. The subretinal blood should also be evacuated carefully, othefwise it can be the starting point for development of subretinal proliferations.

With the discussion of the inner evacuation of the subretinal fluid and the necessary retinotomy we have arrived at the problem of the retinal surgery.

Surgical treatment of the retina was unthinkable for various reasons and belonged to the forbidden themes, similarly as the vitreous surgery before the open sky vitrectomy. Retinal surgery was practically never necessary in the conventional detachment surgery. Later, when the difficult forms of retinal detachment started to be treated with pars plana vitrectomy, for the first time a neccssity appeared in many situations to complete the vitrectomy with retinal surgery. But the problem of closing the hole, particularly in the posterior pole, with the immobile and contracted retina, presented itself even more sharply and warned to caution. A strong mental barrier that always exists at passing such borders was also the reason that very few surgeons dared to take that step. Only the security of the postoperative silicone oil tamponade made this step possible first mentally and then technically. Although in the use of the original Scott's technique carrying out of the retinotomy was possible, because of lack of the vitrectomy and other advantages of the bimanual technique, it was an intervention with uncertain result, which was carried out only in utmost need. Only with the use of bimanual pars plana vitrectomy and its further development in combination with the silicone injection it was possible to develop and apply the retinal surgery to the full extent. The treatment of cases more and more difficult brought us repeatedly in the situation in which we had to recognize the limits of vitrectomy. The removal of the vitreous and the fibrotic tissue was insufficient in the most difficult cases when the retina itself was shrunk, shortened or incarcerated. The cutting, removing and subsequently fixing the retina appeared necessary and promising in such cases. For 6 years the retinal surgery has been performed with us systematically and as routine in a great number of patients. In this way it has become an important part of the surgical concept without which the treatment of the most difficult cases is totally unimaginable. In this relatively long time we have become acquainted not only with advantages but also with risks and complications of this surgery and we have learnt that it may be used only under strict observation of certain principles and rules. Before we start to discuss these principles in particular, we would like, although it seems superfluous at the first sight, to make a few general remarks concerning the retina.

The retina is, as well known, a highly developed tissue, in which the function ability is not equally divided from the anatomical and physiological point of view. Already in the conventional surgery, for decades, the peripheral part of the retina is destroyed, though not always consciously. The performing of the surgical retinotomy and retinectomy in the periphery is not a revolutionary intervention in the functional sense either. The idea of amputation of a less important part and preservation of the more important ones, which was always a basic surgical idea, has always been present in retinal surgery. The whole manipulation with the retina during or after the retinal surgery, which is frequently very extensive, is relatively well tolerated by the retina as a tissue with regard to later recovery of the function. These facts make the mystification of the retina as tissue superfluous and at the same time the retinal surgery real and possible. The nature of the proliferative process makes this, in itself destructive and amputating surgery, unfortunately, also necessary.

The decision to apply the retinal surgery in a single case has, for various reasons, to be made with great caution. Employment of the retinal surgery in the operative procedure is an irreversible step that has not only immediate consequences for the course of the operation but can also, under circumstances, influence the postoperative course.

The mobility of the retina during surgery is at first only to estimate after removal of the vitreous and the epiretinal membranes. A preceding retinotomy will make this estimation impossible and the later removal of the epiretinal membranes very difficult. The retinectomy of the incarcerated retina, as a rule, will turn much bigger if it is done before removal of the membranes.

So there are many more examples which can prove that the use of retinal surgery at a wrong moment can negatively influence the whole course of the operation. Further reasons can be found in the postoperative course. The remaining epiretinal membranes will proliferate very soon after the operation, even before scars after retinopexy are formed. The reproliferation of these membranes has serious consequences if it occurs at the edge of the cut retina.

Let us remark in the end that retinal surgery represents a considerable and additional trauma, which brings in the eye new elements (blood, debris) for provocation of the proliferation. These reasons should warn us to use retinal surgery only as the last remedy and at the right moment. For this purpose it seems useful to set some basic rules for the use of retinal surgery: (1) a preoperative decision to apply retinal surgery is in most cases not possible and even not necessary; (2) decision should take place during the operation and has to be done after the overall view and the estimation of the entire situation; (3) employment of the retinal surgery basically occurs only after removal of the vitreous and the epiretinal membranes; (4) retinotomy and retinectomy should fundamentally be performed with great reserve the more one moves from the periphery to the centre of the retina; one should try to keep intact as much of the central retina as possible; (5) careful and as atraumatic as possible surgery is the law of the first order, removal of the debris after retinotomy is very important.

After setting the basic rules, the employment of retinal surgery in particular situations will be described thoroughly.

The size and the place of retinotomy is completely dependent on its purpose. Small retinotomy will mostly be used, as already described, at endodrainage. Further it will also be necessary at removal of local subretinal proliferations and at removal of small quantities of silicone oil behind the retina.

Large limbus parallel retinotomy is mostly performed in the farthest periphery and serves to loosening the traction in the shortened retina. Removal of massive subretinal proliferations and large quantities of silicone oil behind the retina are further indications for a large peripheral retinotomy.

Radial retinotomy has not so many indications and has to be carried on with much more caution and reserve. Instead of small radial retinotomies which are propagated at contracted edges of giant tears it is much better to remove the whole edge of the tear. It has to be strongly warned against large radial retinotomies in the circularly shortened and contracted retina. With cutting, the retina contracts further and that leaves a large area of bare pigment epithelium and curled edges of the cut retina. Only with peripheral and locally circular retraction of the retina the radial retinotomy is well advised.

Retinectomy or cutting out and removing of the retina is fundamentally used for three purposes. First, in situations where the adherent membranes cannot be peeled off from the retina, the retina is removed together with the membranes. The avital, not functioning retina should also be removed and this is the second purpose of retinectomy. The last indication is cutting the retina from the places, mostly proliferation scars, where the retina is incarcerated.

For removal of subretinal proliferations, which are often difficult to estimate through the retina and therefore frequently underestimated, two rules should be valid. First, it is certain that not every subretinal strand has to be removed. After cleaning of the retina and after the endodrainage the retina has to be examined for its mobility. If it comes out that the subretinal strands are not the cause of detachment they should be left alone. The second rule is that a large peripheral retinotomy is less radical and traumatizing than a small central one, through which we try to pull large subretinal membranes. At the end of such a manipulation mostly a large central hole remains, without certainty that all membranes have been removed. A large retinotomy demands much more work, but it secures a good view at removal of membranes and is much more sparing for the central retina. The small retinotomy should be used centrally in very limited and easily surveyed subretinal proliferations.

The question of surgical retina fixation arises as natural after the discussion on retinal surgery. Various techniques of the retina fixation will be described in detail in the corresponding parts. It should only be said in this place that this, certainly very valuable technique is employed on a much smaller scale than it is generally considered. A retina which is mobile and free of membranes tends itself to attachment and the gentle power of the injected silicone oil is already sufficient to attach it in most cases. In very extreme cases the retina is so changed that it has to be fixed mechanically before the silicone injection.

The retinopexy has an established place in this surgical concept and should be performed at the end of the operation. As for various reasons endodiathermy cannot be used for development of chorioretinal adhesion from inside, cryopexy and light (argon and xenon) coagulation remain as the method of choice. We have almost exclusively used cryopexy in our surgery. It was basically used for the periphery in the whole range of 360° and centrally for the edges of retinal defects.

Besides for the purpose of chorioretinal adhesion we have often employed cryopexy for prevention of proliferation. Our firm clinical impression is that the membrane proliferation is less progressive or fails to appear at all after intensive cryopexy. This impression has yet to be proved experimentally. Cryopexy is mostly performed from inside under control of the microscope. In case of peroperative miosis cryopexy was performed transsclerally.

It seems to us that in future a combination of central endolasercoagulation with peripheral cryopexy will be most helpful.

Finally, the role of diaphragm in this surgical concept should be briefly discussed. An intact iris diaphragm is very important for functioning of the eye in the new situation with silicone oil in the posterior part of the eye. Our experience with surgical midriasis, as the removal of a part of the iris is sometimes called euphemistically, is very negative from our former experience. The mutilated iris was frequently curled backwards, became fibrotic and adherent to other tissue, silicone oil came, at least in the upper part, in contact with the cornea and in this way is the good fundus view, as the only advantage, paid too dearly. After introduction of iridectomy at 6 o'clock the function of the iris as the regulator of iridectomy opening is even more important.

The peroperative miosis at the operation is certainly a very disturbing matter. For the solution of this problem, however, the temporary fixation of the iris should be chosen.

3. Instrumentation

As we have mentioned in the introduction, the new development in the vitreoretinal surgery would be difficult to imagine without the development of new instruments. This part of our work was made much easier by the existence of the instruments workshop in our clinic. Great readiness of the people working there, their inventivity and professional skill, which were always at our disposal, stimulated us to look for new technical solutions. Their instruments have made our daily work much easier and have positively influenced our results in a high degree.

The new instruments, constructed in this way are, on the one hand, improvements of the already existing instruments with which we were not satisfied in our work at that time, or on the other hand, the completely new ones, which at that moment were not to be found for the corresponding purpose.

In the development of the new instruments we have always tried to avoid the construction of complicated, multifunctional and independent instruments. Not only because more than enough such boxes already belong to the basic equipment of our theatre, but also because in our opinion most manipulations can be performed best with simple mechanical instruments. The manipulations which we have to perform in vitreoretinal surgery are really very simple. Picking, cutting, removing or fixing of the tissue are complicated only because they have to be performed in a small space difficult to illuminate and under the water. If we accept that the observation of the operative course and the desired magnification in the observation by means of the microscope and the contact lens are more or less satisfactorily solved, there remain surgical-technically various possibilities for performance of the operation. Instead of trying to 'overmaster' the given situation with the complicated multifunctional instruments we have rather tried to adapt the situation for the use of two instruments with two hands. Therein we have encountered mainly two problems: illumination and presentation of the operation field. Illumination should be in the surgeon's hand as little as possible, as in this way the use of the second instrument is blocked. Presentation of the operation field is, as well-known, particularly difficult with the work in the periphery and with the 12 o'clock position. Both problems with the work in the periphery are solved well with the coaxial microscope light and the scleral indentation. With the work more posteriorly the optimum solution is to be found with the use of four-port system described later. In this way the possibility is created for the use of various small instruments adapted for particular situations and at the same time the use of the vitrectome, compared to the beginning period, is strongly reduced. The cutting power of the vitrectome is mostly used for removal of structures that cannot be gripped (vitreous, blood clots, etc.).

Simultaneously, we have tried to unify the motorized instruments as much as possible (vitrectome and microscissors) with the intention to make their use easier.

In the following paragraphs we shall confine ourselves mainly to the description of the instruments constructed in our workshop, which we use in the operations daily. Beside the technical description we shall say something about the clinical use of the instruments where it seems useful.

Microsurgical system

The microsurgical system is a modification of the original vitrectomy devices by Klöti and O'Malley with which we used to work in the beginning.

This microsurgical system consists of an irrigation-aspiration part and a power supply for vitrectome and microscissors (Fig. 1).

The system works on mainpower and is controlled by a multi-functional footswitch for the following functions:
- irrigation;
- irrigation-suction (linear to preset level);
- cutting;
- cutting-irrigation;
- cutting-irrigation-suction.

The suction of the irrigation-aspiration part can be adjusted up to 500 mm Hg (650 mbar) and is connected to an adjustable venting system to relieve the air to the atmosphere whereby the underpressure within the silicone tubing is stopped and possible residual suction is eliminated. To avoid a slight aspiration which could occur by the height of the infusion bottle, the system has been provided with a time controlled pinch valve so that an ideal venting adjustment can be done. The power supply for the electromagnetically driven vitrectome and microscissors can be set on a frequency from 0–480 cuts/min. Single cutting or closing of the microscissors can be done by one function of the multifunctional footswitch.

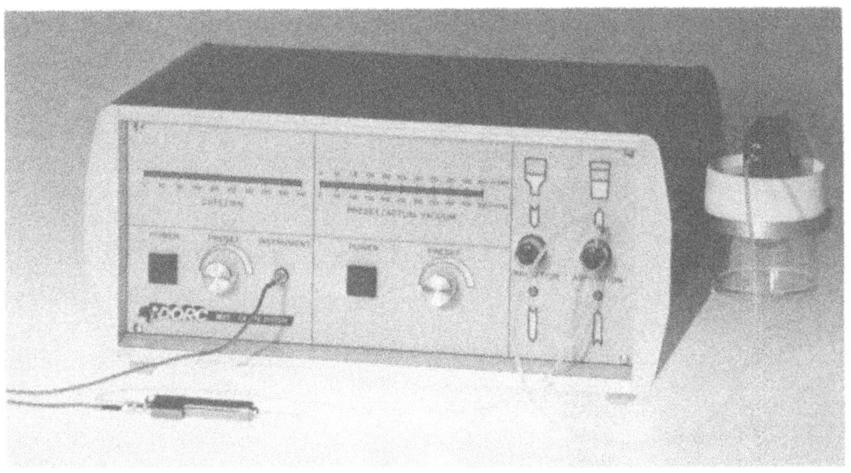

Figure 1.

Vitrectome diameter 0.9 mm (20 gauge)

The vitrectome operates according to an electromagnetic system which gives a guillotine cutting action to the knife (Fig. 2). At the time of the cutting action the inner knife may have a slow rotation of 360°, which prolongs its sharpness. The handpiece itself consists of five parts and is made of titanium. It also has a possibility to adjust the port size from 0–0.9 mm, which can be locked. The dimensions are: length 60 mm, diameter 12 mm, weight 35 g, cutting rate maximum 450/min.

Power controlled vitreous microscissors

The power controlled scissors are working by means of a 6 V electronic controlled electrometer which provides the forward and backward movement of the outer shaft while a three-way footswitch controls the close-open and cutting (Fig. 3).
– Vitreous microscissors straight;
– vitreous microscissors 135°;
– vitreous microscissors with blades at right angle to the shaft.
Except of the 135° microscissors all these scissors have a positive action, which means that the outer shaft moves. The handpiece is partly made of titanium and stainless steel on which same types of vitreous scissors, as with the ergonomic hand-held handles can be mounted.

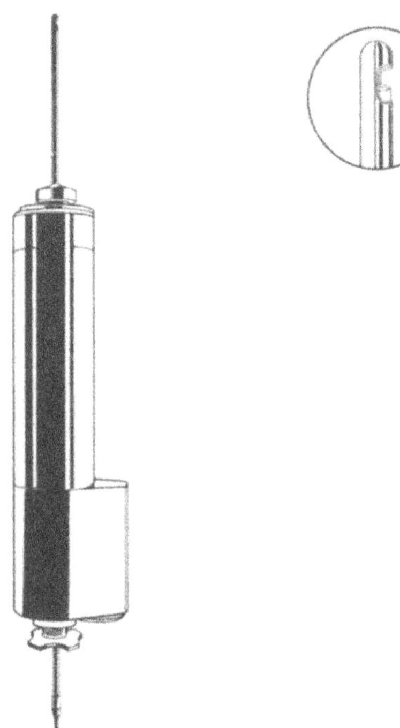

Figure 2.

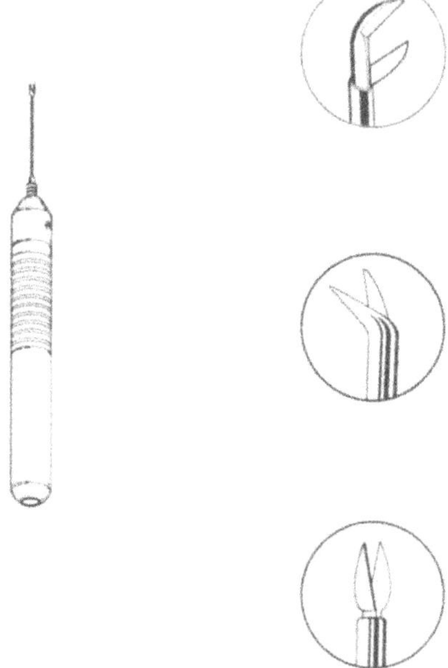

Figure 3.

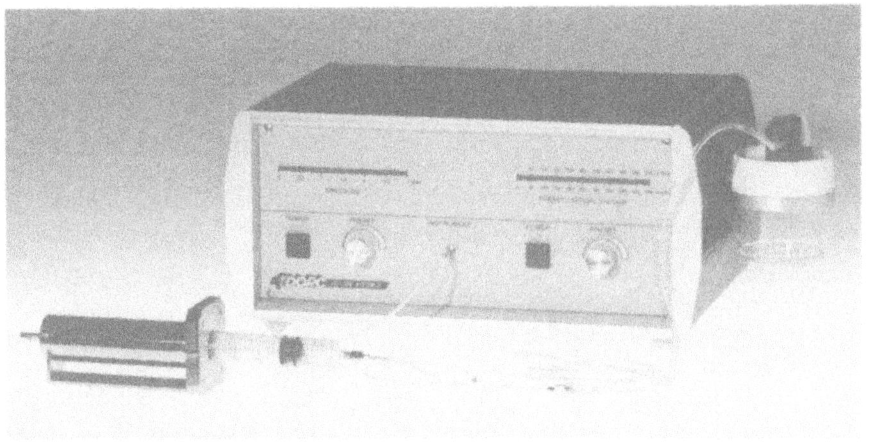

Figure 4.

VFI/VFE Unit (viscous fluid injection/viscous fluid evacuation) was originally designed for the injection and aspiration of silicone oil (Fig. 4). Its injection part has a built-in pressure regulator and an electronic system to control the connected high pressure and the working pressure for the syringe. The aspiration part consists of an electronically controlled system with a built-in vacuum pump which can be adjusted up to 500 mm Hg (650 mbar). Irrigation and aspiration are controlled by a two-way footswitch which also gives the possibility to use both functions at the same time.

VFI holder for 20 cc disposable syringe for silicone oil

The VFI holder consists of a disposable syringe holder with piston and a lock-plate. After closing the lock-plate the 20 cc syringe is securely fixed (Fig. 5). By means of a high pressure tube the syringe holder is connected to the unit. The syringe (with luor-lock connector) is connected with silicone tubing to the infusion plug. To aspirate silicone oil out of the eye we use a disposable aspiration tubing made of polyvinylchloride with luor-lock connectors. It might be possible that different aspiration needles are desired. We use a 0.9 and 1.2 mm aspiration needle with side or end port (Fig. 6).

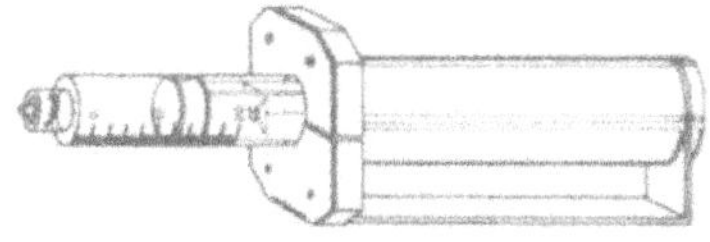

Figure 5.

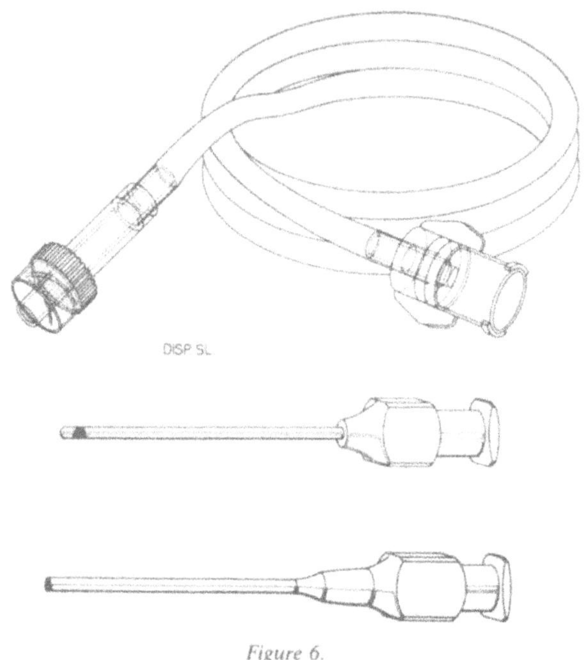

Figure 6.

Module selector

The module selector is connected to the microsurgical system, VFI/VFE unit, diathermy unit and cryo unit. By means of buttons on the front panel of the unit one can choose what kind of unit has to be used, using the same footswitch as for all other units. This avoids working with all types of different footswitches, which might cause confusion during surgery.

Infusion plug forceps

The infusion plug forceps has a length of 115 mm. The gripping part has a diameter of 3 mm, which fits exactly around the silicone infusion tubing and makes the manipulation of the infusion plug very easy (Fig. 7).

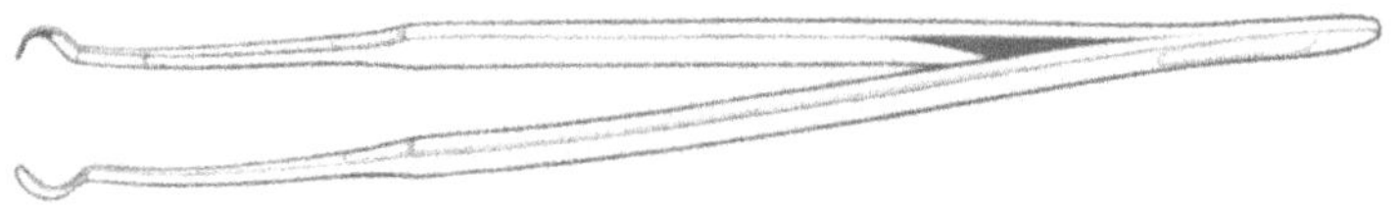

Figure 7.

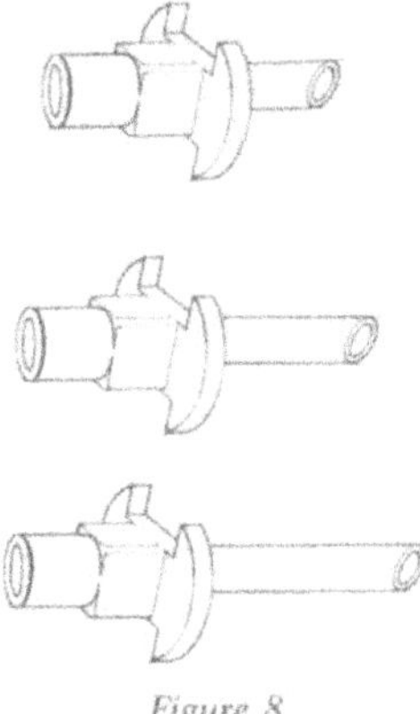

Figure 8.

Infusion plugs diameter 0.9 mm (20 gauge)

The infusion plugs are available in three sizes 3.5, 5 and 7 mm. The suture flanges for securing the plug to the sclera are 4.5 mm long and 2 mm wide (Fig. 8).

Silicone infusion plug

This special infusion plug has a 5 mm long 19 gauge (1 mm) tube with an inner diameter of 0.8 mm. The flanges and the materials are the same as the normal infusion plugs (Fig. 9).

Scleral plug forceps

The scleral plug forceps is made with a cross-action. It has a special tip for insertion and removal of the scleral plugs. The total length is 100 mm (Fig. 10).

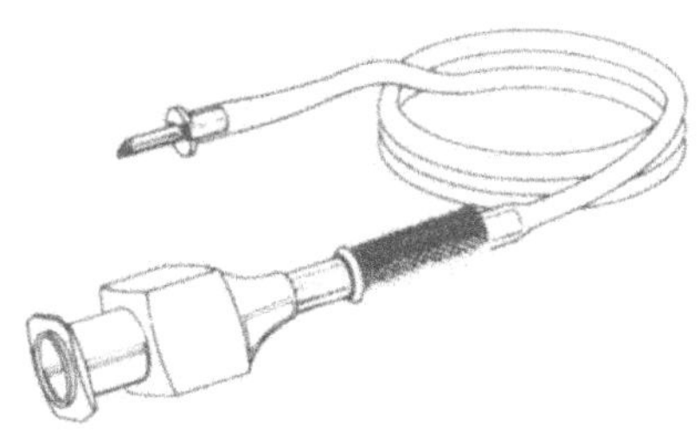

Figure 9.

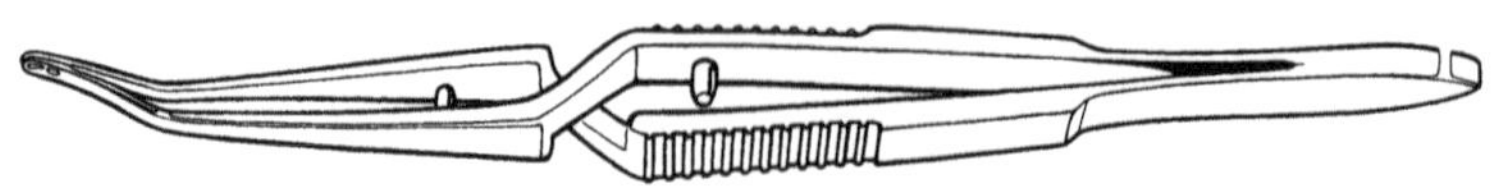

Figure 10.

Scleral plug

The scleral plug is 3 mm long, while the diameter of the knob of the plug is 2 mm. Its penetrating shaft is made of airtight/watertight closures of 20 gauge (0.9 mm) scleral incisions and is made a little conical to provide a better fixation in the sclera (Fig. 11).

Kilp surgical contact lens

The lens is made of quartz glass and has an optical window with a diameter of 9.5 mm. A silicone ring, with a diameter of 14 mm and with the same curve as the contact lens, provides a perfect fixation on the eye and prevents the air bubbles between lens and eye (Fig. 12).

The membrane peeler (Fig. 13) is a blunt instrument which, among other things, is therefore suitable for explorative work among retinal folds, where one often has to separate the retina from the membranes without good visibility. A further possibility is to use the back of the instrument for retinal 'massage' of the contracted retina. The stainless steel handle of the membrane peeler has a diameter of 3 mm and has a length of 90 mm (the same handle is used with the membrane spatula and scratcher). Its 20 gauge chrome-nickel tip is 33 mm long and has a round end, while just behind the top a 4 mm long recess

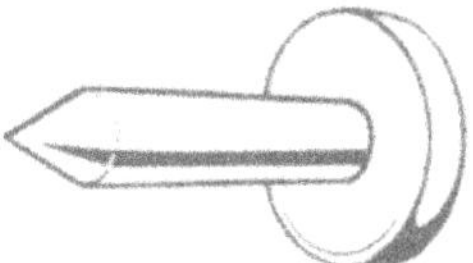

Figure 11.

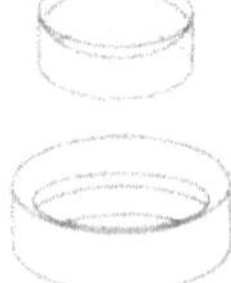

Figure 12.

30

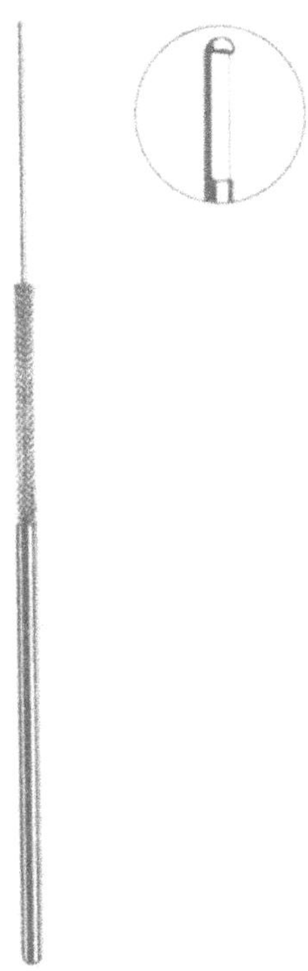

has been made. To prevent reflextions during surgery the tip has a glass peeled finish.

The membrane spatula hooked (Fig. 14) is very suitable for bimanual work, e.g. separating of fibrovascular membranes from the retina. A further possibility is separating of subretinal membranes from the retinal surface by means of retinotomy. The tip is made of 20 gauge (0.9 mm) chrome-nickel steel and is about 33 mm long. Its flatted end is 8 mm long and 0.2 mm thick, while it is bent at an angle of 35° at 5 mm from the top.

The membrane spatula knife (Fig. 14) is also suitable for bimanual work and separating of the fibrotic membranes which are very adherent. Only the thickness of the tip is 0.12 mm and it has very sharp edges to provide the cutting action.

The membrane spatula curved (Fig. 15) is a versatile instrument used in various situations in membrane peeling. Its only difference is the curved top at an angle of 45°, instead of the 8 mm straight angled tip of the spatula hooked.

31

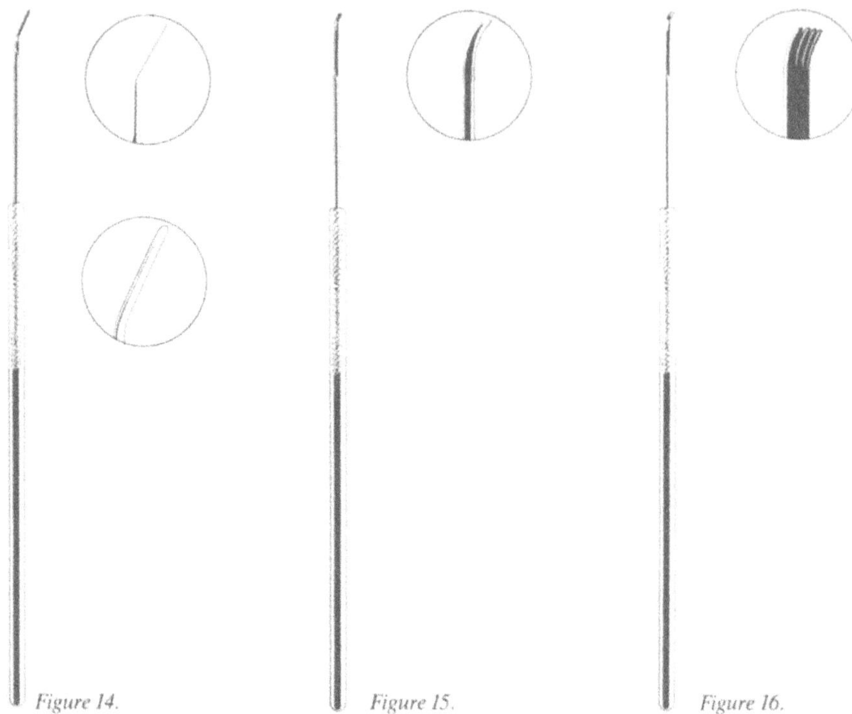

Figure 14.   Figure 15.   Figure 16.

The membrane scratcher (Fig. 16) is used in cleaning of the retina from the structures which are difficult or impossible to grip. It can also be used as a hook to lift the membrane edge. The straight 45° angled top has four small teeth of 0.15 mm wide and 0.4 mm long.

Various *intraocular forcepses* are used to grip and to remove various structures (Fig. 17).

The end gripping forceps and end gripping forceps with micro jaws are mainly used to grip fine structures from the retinal surface. They can also be used in various other situations.

The *forceps with serrated jaws* is very useful in the removal of the material with coarse structure.

The *curved forceps*, which is a modification of the B. Morris forceps has the same jaws and serves for gripping and removing of subretinal proliferations under the retina through a peripheral retinotomy (Fig. 18).

32

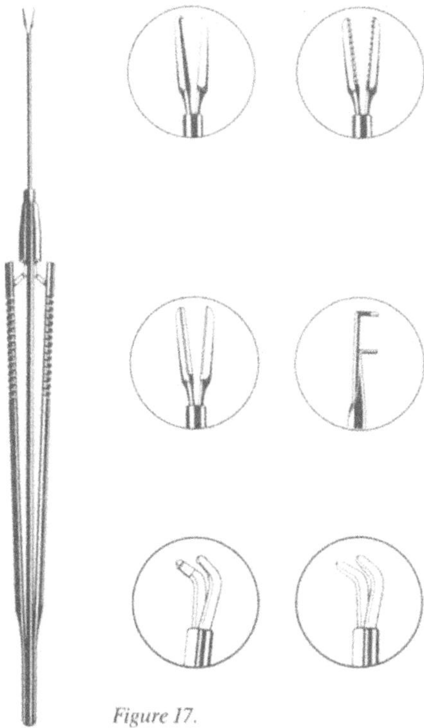

Figure 17.

The *side gripping forceps* is relatively seldom used, but it is useful in gripping of the membranes on the edge of the buckle.

The *forceps with silicone cover* is useful in gripping and removing of foreign bodies and smooth material.

Pick forceps, which is a modification of the McCuen instrument, and *hockey stick forceps* are often used and are useful in various situations in membrane peeling as peeling and gripping instruments.

All these forcepses have a light weight ergonomic stainless steel handle for 360° rotation and easy manoeuvrability. They have a 20 gauge (0.9 mm) shaft and smooth surface for easy entry through the pars plana sclerotomy.

Vitreous scissors

As with the motorised scissors, we also make use of three different types of mechanical scissors (Fig. 19).

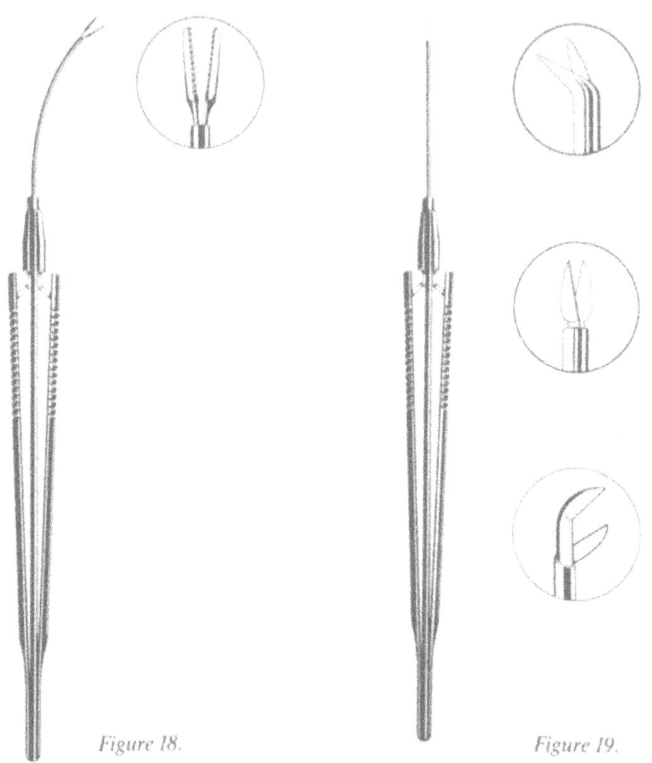

Figure 18. Figure 19.

The vitreous scissors with blades at right angle are very often used in various situations.

The scissors 135° are much used in separation of membranes from the retina in diabetic traction detachment.

The straight scissors are rarely used, but they are very useful in the work in the periphery in the ROP cases.

All these scissors have a light weight ergonomic stainless steel handle for 360° rotation and easy manoeuvrability. They have a 20 gauge (0.9 mm) shaft and smooth surface for easy entry through the pars plana sclerotomy. Except with the 135° scissors the outer tube will move forward and backward while the scissors are standing still. The 135° microscissors have a movable inner blade and a fixed outer blade.

The retinal tack serves for transvitreal fixation of the retina. Its use is described at length in the clinical part of the book. The tack is made of 0.8 mm remanium

34

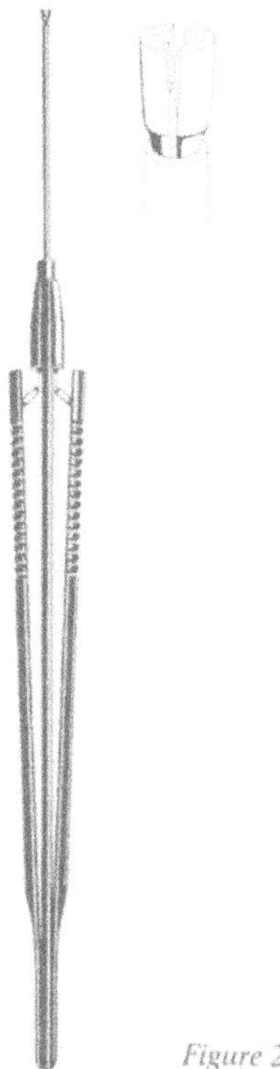

chrome-nickel steelwire. Its perforated needle is 2.5 mm long and has a diameter of 0.3 mm (Fig. 20). The part which will fit in the tack-forceps has a length of 0.7 mm and a diameter of 0.55 mm while the total length of the tack is 3.5 mm.

Retina tack forceps: the handle of the forceps is made of stainless steel with a diameter of 5 mm, while its total length is, including the 20 gauge tip, about 150 mm. Its fixed 20 gauge gripping part can be closed by the movable 20 gauge outer shaft, which gets its action by pressing the handle. The hollow gripping part has the same measures as the retinal tack to provide an exact grip (Fig. 21).

The back-flush needle is a modification of the Charles flute needle. With this modification the greatest disadvantage of the original instrument is removed, namely not functioning of the instrument in sucking of the loose material or the retina. By sliding of a silicone tubing on the needle expressing of the material or the sucked retina is possible with pressing by the finger on the tubing. Fixing of different cannulas on the instrument enables endodrainage of the subretinal

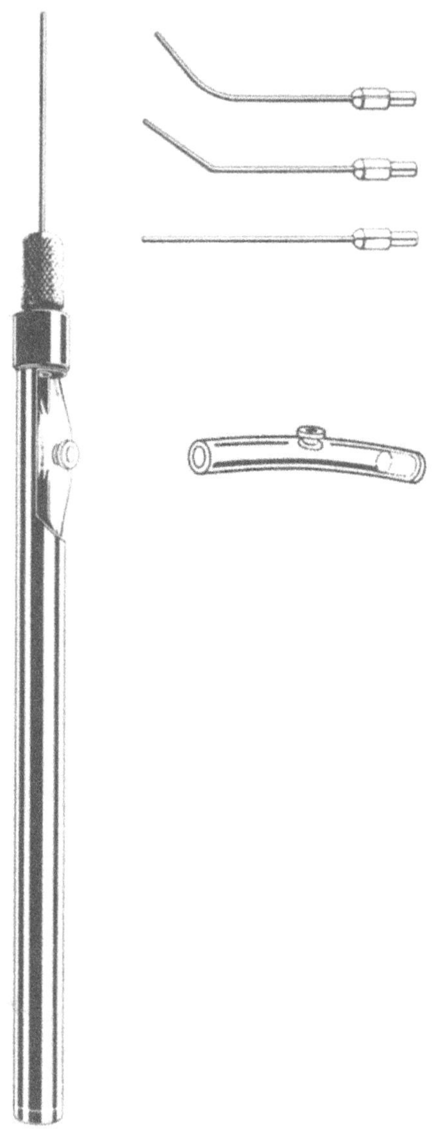

fluid from the periphery. With the curved cannula it is e.g. possible to drain the subretinal fluid through a peripheral retinotomy on the buckle under the central retina (Fig. 22). The instrument consists of a 7 mm round and 112 mm long stainless steel handle, whereby in the middle a small piece of silicone tubing with an exit port is connected to the needle. It is possible to use different types of needles and it is very easy to change the silicone tubing.

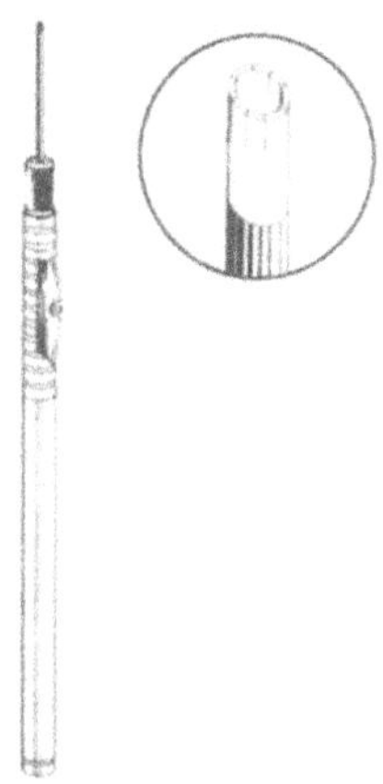

Figure 23.

A further modification is the *brush – back-flush needle*. With the silicone tubing at the end of the needle one can 'clean' the retinal surface very easily and atraumatically and at the same time suck off and remove the material (Fig. 23). The brush needle has to be placed in the original back-flush handpiece. It consists of a 20 gauge 0.89 mm needle and 33 mm long with a 23 gauge (6.6 mm) tip. A thin sleeve of silicone tubing is slided over this tip, which is approximately 0.5 mm longer. This extending silicone sleeve has been cut in eight equal incisions, whereby a sort of brush is created, which can aspirate at the same time.

The combination of the *back-flush needle* and *diathermy* proves its worth in profuse bleedings, where one can simultaneously suck off the blood and coagulate the bleeding site without losing time on exchange of instruments (Fig. 24). The back-flush bipolar diathermy needle is a modified back-flush needle with a fixed 20 gauge needle instead of interchangeable needles and is

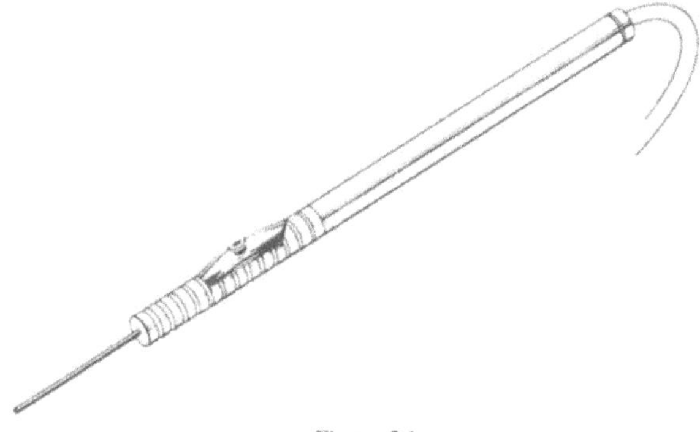

Figure 24.

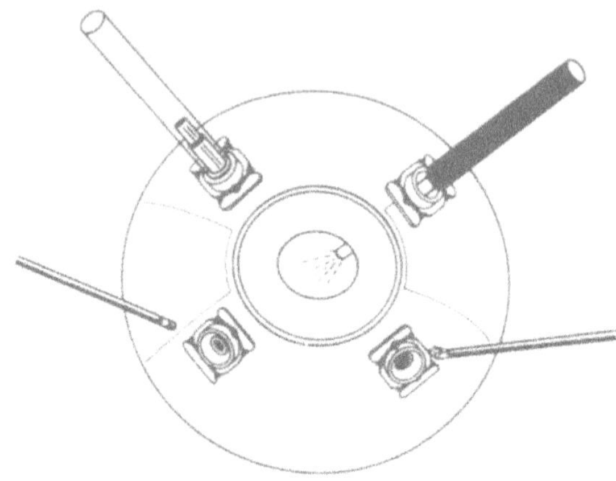

mounted in such a way that it is easy to change the silicone pressure part. The needle itself consists of two insulated capillary tubes, the inner one acting as the positive electrode. As a power source a DORC or Mira diathermy control unit may be used or any source with the same specifications. The back-flush bipolar diathermy needle is made of stainless steel and 112 mm long and has a diameter of 7 mm.

The four-port system is constructed to overcome various disadvantages of the (already) classical vitrectomy technique. By introduction of an independent light source, which gives enough light for most situations, the possibility is created for proper bimanual work. Owing to complete exchangeability there is also the possibility to have illumination and infusion in any desired position, which also means that one can work bimanually from underneath i.e. from 4

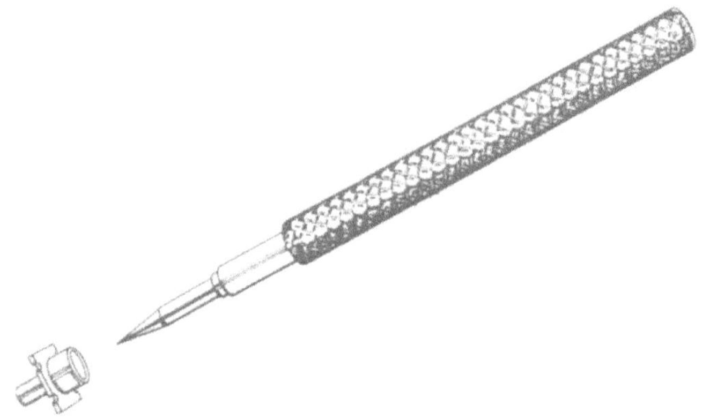

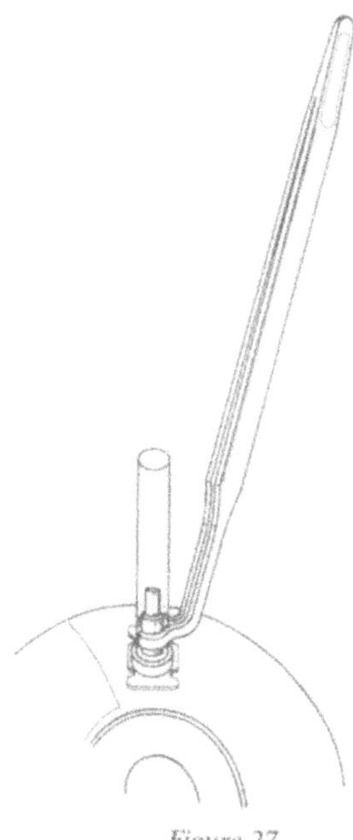

Figure 27.

and 8 o'clock position as well. In this way even the position at 12 o'clock, difficult until now, becomes easy to reach. The whole system is watertight due to the silicone ring and can, when necessary, also at the exchange of instruments, be closed with special plugs. Disadvantages of four, a little larger sclerotomies and of additional work are, particularly in difficult cases, amply overcome by the described advantages (Fig. 25). The cannula of the four-port system is made of stainless steel and consists of a 3 mm long and 1.55 mm outer diameter while the inner diameter of the tube is 1.4 mm. Two flanges for suturing and a silicone ring, for better manoeuvrability and airtight/watertight closure of the cannula when instruments are inserted, are also a part of the cannula (Fig. 26). The silicone ring is also a part of a locking system and can be closed with a special plug. Little rings mounted on the tubes of infusion plugs and special fibre in combination with the silicone ring give a very good and easy fixation of these accessories (Fig. 27).

Beside the described instruments let us mention, for the sake of completeness, that in our daily work we make use of the usual machines for diathermy and cryopexy. As the source of illumination in most operations the Xenon light source is used, which guarantees excellent light conditions during the operation.

Since a very short time we use the endolaser for photo coagulation at the end of the operation.

4. Physical properties of silicone oil

Ever since Cibis first introduced silicone oil (SO) intraocularly to treat complicated retinal detachment (1962), polydimethylsiloxane (PDMS) has been
practically the only silicone oil used for this purpose. Reports on intraocular
application of other types of SO, e.g. fluorinated SO or phenyl SO, are few,
and the results are still inconclusive.

PDMS is produced by the polymerization of oligodimethylsiloxane mole-
cules, each of which contains some dimethylsiloxane units (Fig. 1). While
PDMS exhibits a number of invariable properties (Fig. 2), its molecular weight
(MW) and viscosity* can be altered by varying the length of its polymer chain.

The gelchromatogram in Fig. 3 shows the MW distribution of a typical
PDMS; the average MW of 15,000 determines the viscosity of 1,000 mPa's. By
adjusting the polymerization process to increase or reduce MW, oils of different viscosity can be produced, e.g. a PDMS with an average MW of 30,000
and a viscosity of 5,000 mPa's.

Another way of varying viscosity is to mix two different PDMSs; this results
in an intermediate viscosity corresponding to the newly created average MW.
This is reflected in a quite asymmetrical distribution of MWs (Fig. 4), meaning
that PDMSs of equal viscosity are fully capable of having different MW
distributions.

The polymerization of SO is a chemical process which leads to a statistical
distribution of the length of the polymerized molecules and in that way their
MW. The molecules range from a large number of mean MW to a lesser
number with low molecular weight (LMW) and an even much smaller with
higher MW.

MW distribution can be measured either by gelchromatograms or by testing
for volatility. The first method is precise but difficult; the second yields less
specific information, but is appreciably easier to do.

---

* Dynamic viscosity: mPa's (old term: centipoise); cinematic viscosity: mm²/s (old term: cen-
tistoke).

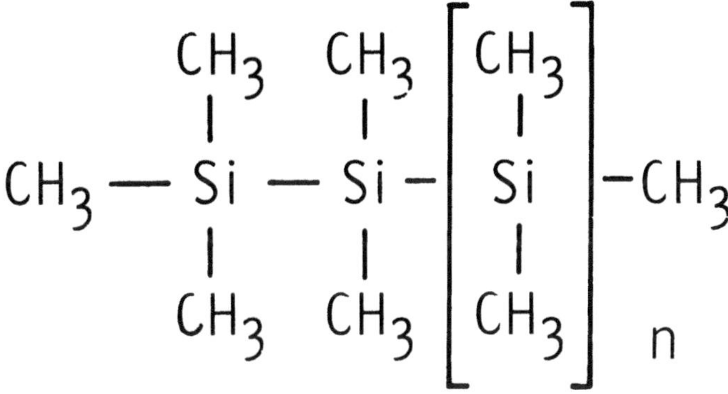

Figure 1. Chemical structure of PDMS.

In the latter procedure SO is kept at 200– C for 24 h, at the end of which time loss in weight is measured. The smaller the molecules the greater the volatility, so that volatility serves as an indicator of the smallest molecules in a given volume.

Moreover, temperatures of 200°C can cause some molecular decomposition, leading to smaller silicone molecule fragments; the volatility test can therefore also serve as a measure of the stability of PDMS.

The gelchromatogram in Fig. 3 shows that while the majority of the PDMS molecules have a high MW, others with a lower MW (<2,400) are present as well. These lower molecular weight components (LMWC) are present either in the linear form of oligodimethylsiloxane units (MW~800–2,400) or, in smaller ring-shaped cyclosiloxanes (MW~300–800), e.g. octamethyl-cyclotetrasiloxane (Fig. 5). They are more frequent in silicone oils with LMW respectively viscosity than in those with higher MW respectively viscosity.

The LMWC can diffuse as vapor out of a silicone bubble in the vitreous cavity into surrounding tissues of the eye (Kampik, 1987). Once diffused, they

refractive index   1. 404

spec. gravity $0.97 \, g/cm^3$ at 25^0 C

surface tension   21 mN/m against air

40 mN/m against water

Figure 2. Invariable properties of PDMS.

41

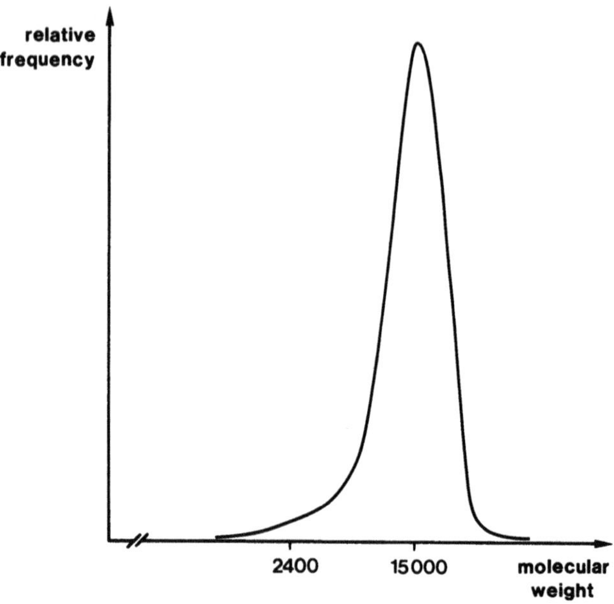

Figure 3. Gelchromatogram of PDMS.

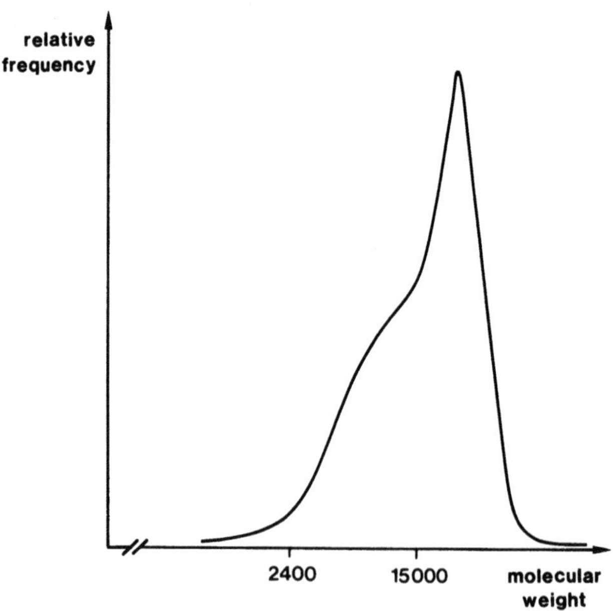

Figure 4. Gelchromatogram of PDMS, mixture of two different SOs.

42

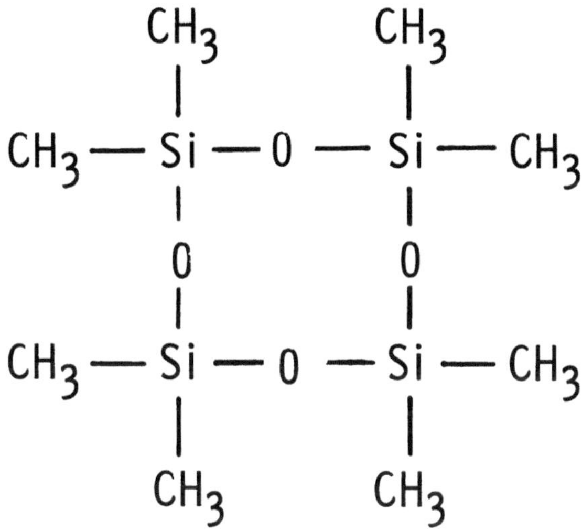

Figure 5. Chemical structure of octamethylcyclotetrasiloxane.

accumulate and recondense into silicone droplets, e.g. in the anterior chamber. This diffusion is best known (Refojo, 1985) for octamethylcylotetrasiloxane, a cyclosiloxane with a MW of 296. This silicone retains a vapor pressure of 2.5 mm Hg at 37° C, suggesting a relatively high diffusion rate, whereas molecules with a MW between 800 and 2,400 display no measurable vapor pressure at 37° C. It is conceivable, however, that even such 'larger' molecules, given a long enough exposure time, might also diffuse into surrounding tissue. This diffusion in the eye is termed 'thermodiffusion' because it is dependent upon the temperature gradient between the anterior and posterior segments of the eye.

Another mechanism leading silicone oil droplets to accumulate in the anterior chamber is emulsification. It results when the normal immiscibility of silicone oil and intraocular fluid due to interface tension (40 mN/m) is overcome by surface active agents or by mechanical forces such as shaking. Eye movements are normally not violent enough to disrupt interface tension and cause emulsification. However, it has recently been shown (Crips, 1986) that both protinaceous substances in the human serum and phospholipids from red blood cells can cause emulsification by weakening the interfacial tension through their bipolar properties. This sequence of events was shown in vitro to be more pronounced in SOs with lower viscosity and those containing LMWC.

In addition of LMWC, it is possible that catalytic remnants left over from the polymerization of PDMS may interact with biological structures in the eye, prompting irritation and undesirable cell reactions. Even though these cata-lysts are inactivated at the end of the polymerization process, there is still no conclusive proof that such interactions between inactivated catalysts and biological tissue do not take place. Since catalystic remnants are ionic in nature, volume resistivity is a good measure of their presence.

Conclusions

Low LMWC and the absence of catalytic remnants cannot presently be viewed conclusively as causes of a better intraocular tolerance considerations supported by clinical and histopathological observations. However, it seems clear that LMWCs are of great importance for the biocompatibility of PDMS and should be avoided at all costs, either by using a silicone oil of very high viscosity or, better, by using PDMS which has been specially prepared so as to eliminate LMWC.

Purified silicone oil has been available in the free market for the last few years. From 1978, when we started working with silicone oil, we have used silicone oil which was not made for medical use and at that time was the only available, namely General Electric SF 96, viscosity 1,000 mPa's with relatively small LMWC (1.5%).

5. Surgical techniques

Different pathoanatomic indication groups demand by their different etiological background also the appropriate surgical techniques. For this reason the surgical technique is described separately with each indication group. To avoid repetition, common phases of the surgical technique (lensectomy, vitrectomy of the vitreous base, etc.) are described in detail in the discussion of the first group – the idiopathic retinal detachment with PVR. The very specific techniques, although they may, incidentally, be used in all groups, are described with the group in which they are used most frequently (e.g. retina fixation with giant tears).

In the description of surgical techniques the regular course of the operation is described.

Difficulties that can develop during the operation and technical solutions by which they are removed are described in the chapter on peroperative complications. In the description of the surgical technique the attempt has been made not to go deeper in generally known technical details of the pars plana vitrectomy and to mention it only as far as it is relevant for a specific surgical technique.

In the performance of operations mostly the instruments designed at our clinic were used. In the description of the technique these instruments are also mentioned where necessary, which does not mean that the same cannot be done with other, similar instruments.

Idiopathic retinal detachment with PVR

As already mentioned, the indenting technique with purpose to release traction or to close the hole has no place any more in our surgical concept. Placing an encircling band serves much better to a better visibility and marking of the retinal periphery during the surgery. The encircling band is placed in previously not operated patients at approximately 12 mm from the limbus as the first step of the operation. A silicone rod of 1 mm diameter is fixed to the sclera in four quadrants and definitely pulled up and tightened so that a mild indentation is achieved. In preoperated eyes the pre-existing encircling band is mostly not revised. The pre-existing radial buckle is mostly removed during the operation. The encircling band is left in its place if it does not strongly indent the bulbus. In this case it is only cut. Removal of radial buckles and transection of the encircling band in the extreme indentation is useful, because every extreme indentation that disturbs the geometry of the inner eye makes removal of membranes and later unfolding of the retina more difficult. This intervention does not take much time and is not traumatizing either. The whole revision of the pre-existing buckle is, on the other hand, not only sometimes very time-consuming and traumatizing, but can in repeatedly operated eyes lead to unnecessary complicatons. Only very seldom is this of any use.

After insertion of the infusion line and performance of two sclerotomies removal of the lens follows. If ever possible it should be done through pars plana. With a Sato knife or a similar instrument the lens is perforated equatorially through both sclerotomies. With the same instrument the lens nucleus is destroyed as much as possible without further damaging the lens capsule. Removal of the lens is performed with the vitrectome or the phako instrument, if possible in the capsule. It is very important not to open the anterior capsule too early and to provoke in this way collapsing of the anterior chamber with subsequent miosis (Fig. 1). After removal of the lens nucleus first the posterior and then the anterior capsule of the lens is removed. After this phase there are still the equatorial remnants of the capsule with zonula fibre behind the iris. These should best be removed with an endgripping forceps around all quadrants (Fig. 2). To secure a better view behind the iris, the corresponding area is indented with a cotton swab. After manual removal of the capsule and zonula the remaining zonula fibres are removed with the vitrectome. Attention should be paid not to damage the ciliary body. The whole procedure of removal of the lens can occur very well under the coaxial light of the microscope and without contact lens.

In this way it is practically possible to remove, with the vitrectome, all lenses, even in patients above 60. On lenses with a hard nucleus it will be possible to operate with a phako instrument. However, there are always a few lenses which have to be operated ab externo. A great disadvantage of this combined operation is a fresh corneal wound in the later phase of the operation, if e.g. after the silicone oil injection one has to operate some time with changing intraocular pressure and frequently with high pressure. Bursting of the wound and iris prolaps are frequently its unpleasant consequences. To avoid this to a certain extent, after introducing infusion and making of scleral openings the eye should be opened with a corneal incision of 90°. The anterior

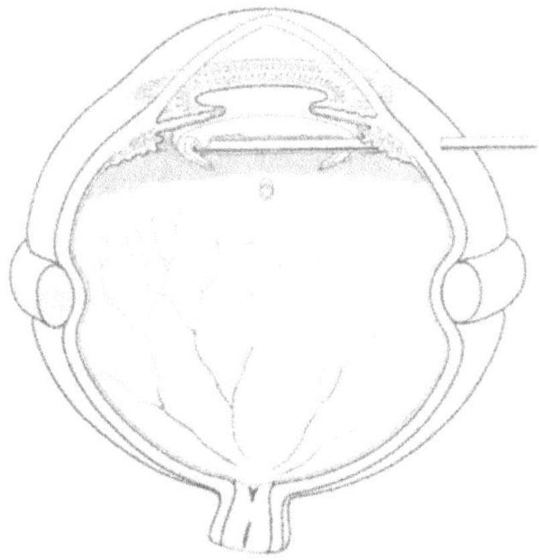

Figure 1. Removal of the lens.

capsule should be opened with the Sato knife through pars plana and the nucleus expressed through a small corneal opening. After hermetical closing of the wound the capsule remnants and zonula should be removed in the above-mentioned way.

The direct disadvantage of the whole manipulation is the narrow pupil developed in this way. In most cases the pupil is dilated again after 10–15 min if the infusion has contained adrenalin from the beginning. With a persisting miosis, a surgical dilation of the pupil with temporary iris sutures should be performed.

Removal of the lens can be performed as a rule at the beginning of the operation. However, there are sometimes cases in which in the beginning one hesitates whether to use silicone oil, and perhaps will end the operation with a gas injection. In such cases removal of the clear lens is not necessary and the decision whether to remove the lens can be brought after vitrectomy and assessment of the status of the retina.

After removal of the lens it is advisable to re-examine the fundus thoroughly. In the periphery this should be done with indenting. The connections of the retina with the shrunk vitreous and the newly developed membranes have to be registered to understand the causes of traction and immobility of the retina. Comprehension and estimation of the given situation is necessary to make a good operative plan. The situation is comparable to a thread ball that has to be unraveled. It is notorious that one should not begin at the wrong end. It does not seem superfluous.to explain the importance of this statement more closely with some examples. In many cases the picture of the fundus is e.g. dominated by epiretinal membranes that immobilize the whole central retina and obstruct the access to the disc. It is very tempting and not very difficult

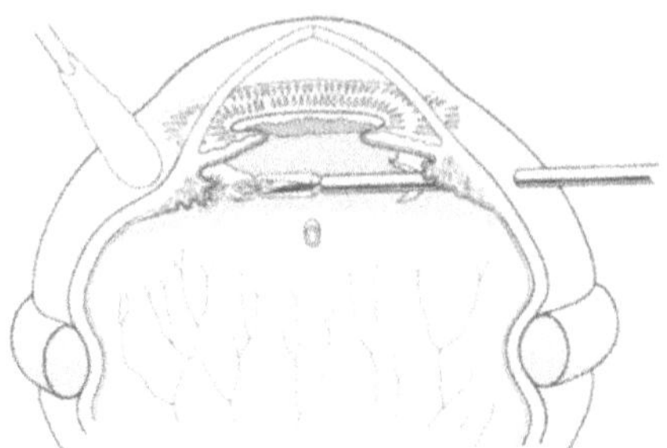

Figure 2. Removal of capsula remnants with the forceps.

either to remove these membranes immediately and to mobilize the retina. But in this way the peripheral retina also becomes more mobile, and removal of epiretinal membranes in the periphery and vitrectomy of the vitreous base become much more difficult. It is much more reasonable to perform the latter first and to benefit from immobility of the retina caused by central membranes. A retinotomy performed in the vicinity of still present epiretinal membranes, to give a simple example, will make removal of membranes later very difficult, if not even impossible. Therefore the retinotomy should always be done following removal of membranes. Further, in very adherent membranes there is a great risk of making an iatrogenic hole. A retinal hole has not so hard consequences in this technique, but if the retina has been torn, removal of membranes is more difficult, because under traction the hole becomes bigger and bigger. Therefore under the circumstances (particularly distinct in diabetic proliferation) it is much better to remove the most difficult membranes at the end.

These and many other examples point out the necessity of planning very clearly. Although it is very difficult, because of great variety of cases, to give fast rules for an operative planning, we would like to try to describe at least some guide-lines. The description of the guide-lines will be introduced with a few explanations of typical pathoanatomical situations.

The given situation is created by a biological process which has set various mechanical forces to work. The play of the mechanical forces is also greatly decided by all pre-existing anatomical relations. To keep this in mind is indispensable for comprehension and interpretation of the pathoanatomical situation.

In most cases of idiopathic retinal detachment with PVR it concerns basically four different mechanisms. The vitreous is mostly detached, shrunk and retracted to the anterior part of the vitreous cavity. By shrinking of the vitreous a circular traction is exercised on the retina in the area of the vitreous base, where the retina strongly adheres to the vitreous. The result of this traction is a retinal detachment with radial folds as far as the posterior pole.

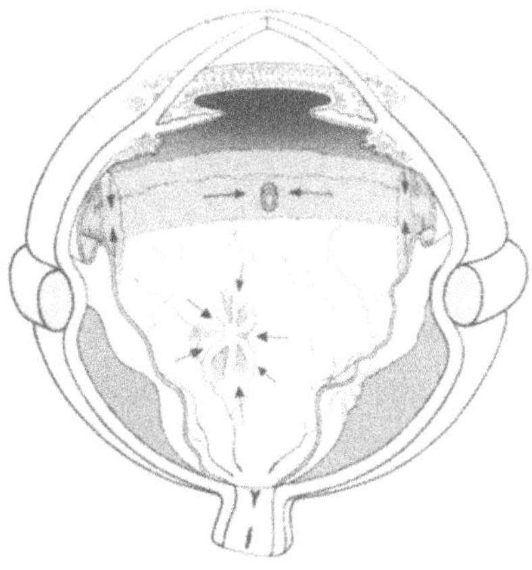

Figure 3. Usual traction mechanisms in PVR detachment.

This process can be, and frequently is, helped by the contraction of the newly developed membranes on the surface of the retina and the back surface of the vitreous. The second mechanical factor is the shrinking of the vitreous in sagital direction, by which the retina is pulled forward in shape of a circular fold (so-called anterior loop traction). As the third factor one should mention tangential traction of the newly developed epiretinal membranes, which, by their contraction, form star-shaped folds (Fig. 3). The last factor is proliferations on the back surface of the retina. They are much more frequent in traumatic retinal detachments, but can sometimes develop after unsuccessful retinal surgery, particularly after subretinal haemorrhages. The retina is then mostly detached in the shape of a 'clothes-line' phenomenon or the subretinal proliferations build a circular formation around the disc (napkin ring).

The pathological changes will, naturally, be different from case to case, because the described factors are present in different quantities and combined with one another in different ways. However, the pathoanatomical picture that we find before surgery is decided by these factors and the operative procedure has to be adapted to this situation. For this reason it is best to begin vitrectomy with removal of the central vitreous. In this way the peripheral retina is circularly relieved to a certain extent and some more work space is created. The central vitreous is mostly easy to remove. If it is strongly fibrotic and tense it is best to cut it first with a Sato knife. As the next step vitrectomy in the vitreous base area is performed. In preoperated eyes with scarred peripheral retina this is relatively simple, but with the detached retina one has to be very careful with the more and more mobile retina, which is by accident easily sucked in the opening of the vitrectome. The vitrectomy of the vitreous base is performed best with scleral depression and without contact glas under coaxial illumination of the microscope (Fig. 4). Very much attention is paid to

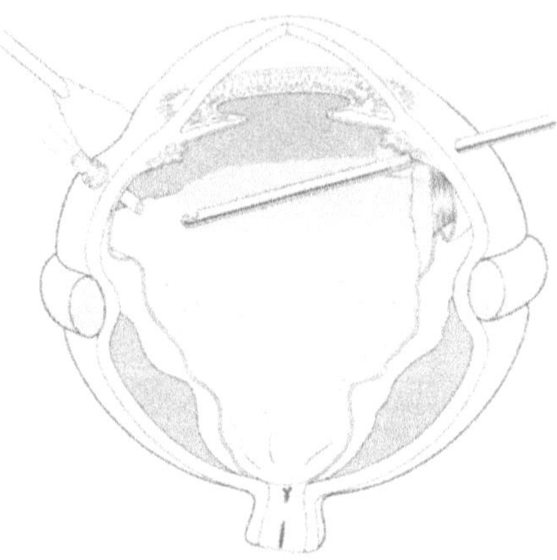

Figure 4. Removal of vitreous in the area of vitreous base with the vitrectome and scleral indentation.

the area of sclerotomy to prevent a later incarceration of the retina by means of residuing vitreous fibres.

Removal of the vitreous in the area of the vitreous base relieves almost completely the sagital traction. The circular traction, which is partly also caused by newly developed membranes, is in this way only partly relieved. The membranes are in equatorial area, frequently connected to degeneration areas and tear flaps. They pass over into the vitreous base and are very difficult to remove with the vitrectome. They often cause radial folding of the equatorial retina. It is easiest to grasp them with the forceps. As they are firmly adherent to the vitreous base and to the retina, there is a great risk of tearing the retina. Working with two hands and two instruments can substantially reduce this risk.

Removal of all membranes can hardly occur without making iatrogenic holes. Nevertheless, on the other hand, leaving the membranes means almost certainly a reproliferation and redetachment. To the most difficult cases belong high myopics, who except many pre-equatorial degeneration areas with vitreous adherence also have a far posterior reaching vitreous base. Besides, the retina is very thin and atrophic in these eyes so that it tears easily. (In extremely difficult cases the retina can be attached only if the whole peripheral retina is removed together with adherent membranes. This can only be done after removal of central membranes and cleaning of the retina (Fig. 5).

When this phase of the operation has been performed with not too much damage for the retina (a few peripheral holes have not bad consequences), removal of the central membranes follows. In the older cases it is not difficult work. If the disc is completely covered with folds and membranes, one goes

50

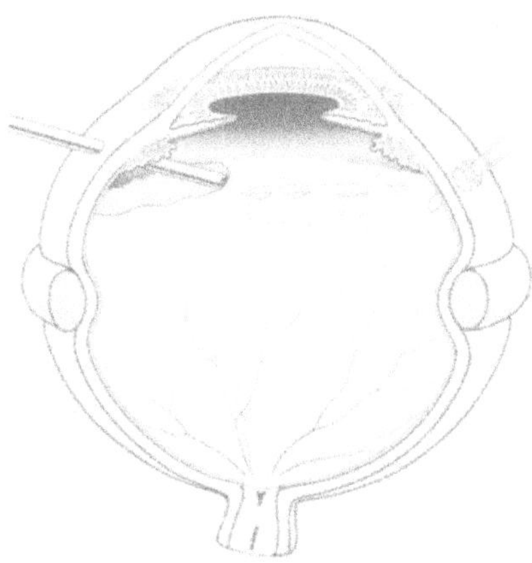

Figure 5. Retinectomy – removal of the retina together with adherent membranes peripheral to the tears.

between the folds with the membrane peeler (with a round back), which cannot damage the retina. Exploring simultaneously, one hooks the membranes and tries to remove them from the retina. Once the membranes are lifted a little from the retina, the instrument is changed. The endgripping – or pick – forceps is taken and the membrane peeled from the retina preferably in one piece. Scissors are not a suitable instrument with it, because one wants to take out the whole membrane and may not leave any pieces of it on the retina surface. With extensive membranes which cover a large part of the retina one can use two instruments – and work under coaxial illumination (Fig. 6).

In fresh cases the situation is more complicated. The changes do not seem so impressive and the retina is relatively mobile. The picture seems much more harmless, but it soon appears to be a deception. The membranes have not matured yet and are in various stages of maturity. The most conspicuous membranes, which often form little starfolds, can be removed without great trouble, because they already contain enough collagen. A short blunt spatula is used and a suitable place found to lift the membrane edge. When an edge is there, the peeling of the membrane is performed with the forceps. It is not advisable to use a curved sharp needle and similar instruments as they may damage the retina too easily.

Real difficulties begin with the membranes that cannot be seen well. Distorted vessels are to be seen, the retina reflex is also typical and points to the existence of a membrane, but it is still invisible. The retina in this area, compared to the other parts, is also a little immobile. If one is resigned to it and removes only visible membranes, the hidden membranes will become visible and active in a few weeks and will certainly cause a redetachment. Removal can be tried with the instrument in the shape of a scratcher with blunt teeth.

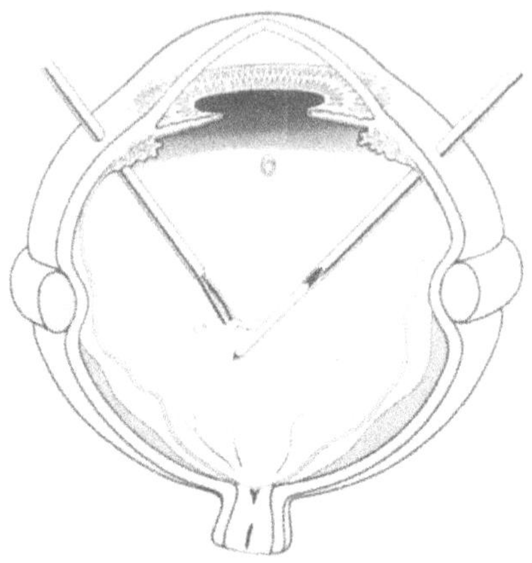

Figure 6. Removal of central epiretinal membranes – technique with two instruments.

The edge of the membranes may be found where the reflex ceases. The found membrane edge is picked up with the forceps. It is sometimes surprising what can be removed yet from the retina surface with a little patience.

Another manifestation of proliferation are pigment clumps deposited on the surface of the retina, which have not yet become membranes. The best instrument is again the scratcher with which one can scratch over the retina without damaging it. Scratched off cells and immature membranes can be easily sucked away with the brush-back-flush needle (Fig. 7). Simultaneously the pigment clumps still attached to the retina can also be removed and sucked away with the silicone brush. The forceps can be used with particles still holding on – frequently along the big vessels.

The three described phases of vitrectomy with membranectomy: vitrectomy of the vitreous base, vitrectomy and membranectomy of the equatorial retina and membranectomy of the central retina serve to mobilize the retina. The mobility of the retina can be judged when the retina is completely free of the vitreous and fibrotic membranes and, which is very important, anatomically almost intact. A few little holes in the periphery or in the centre of the retina will not influence the behaviour of the retina in aqueous environment (only so the mobility can be judged).

Large iatrogenic holes or intentionally made retinotomies will influence the behaviour of the retina so that the judgement on its mobility will become much more difficult.

The judgement of the retina mobility is very important in respect to the right moment of the silicone injection. Only a completely mobile retina can be attached with the silicone oil injection.

The mobility and the behaviour of the retina can be judged most easily with endodrainage. It is best to drain the subretinal fluid through a pre-existing

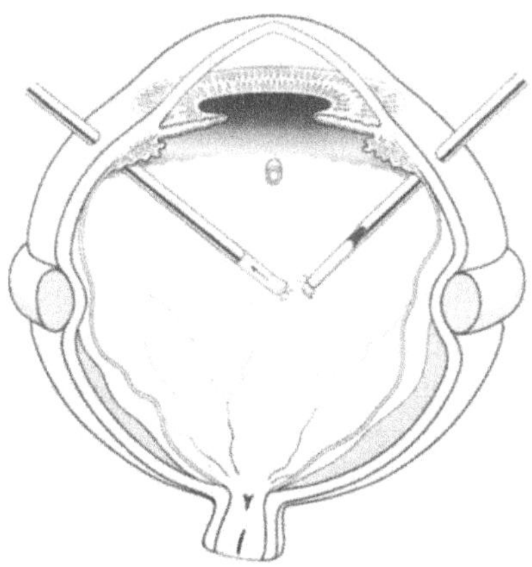

Figure 7. Cleaning of the retina with the scratcher and the brush back-flush needle.

hole. If there is none, a small retinotomy is made, which can be used later, with the silicone injection, for endodrainage. The place of the retinotomy should preferably be in the upper quadrants and far from big vessels and places where there were membranes. After endodiathermy coagulation on the chosen position a little hole in the retina is made with the scissors tip. A back-flush needle with the silicone brush is placed in the hole and the intraocular pressure a little increased. With evacuation of the subretinal fluid it is immediately to be seen how the retina behaves. A retina which is free in all parts and mobile will immediately show tendency to attach. On the contrary, in a contracted retina the power of infusion will not be sufficient to change the position of the retina. (This useful test will not be possible with big retina holes because of unobstructed circulation between the intravitreal and subretinal space.) With this test it can be found out whether silicone oil may be injected or whether further measures to mobilize the retina have to be taken. We want to add yet that this test, besides its usefulness, is easy to perform and (apart from retinotomy) completely harmless. The same cannot be said for fluid-gas exchange. The gas injection forces the retina, which is not harmless, and what is even more important, through its power it can give a deceptive picture of the mobility of the retina.

If with the test a good mobility of the retina has been detected, silicone oil can be injected immediately afterwards. Simultaneously with the silicone injection the intravitreal and subretinal fluid is passively evacuated through the back-flush needle. The mobile retina will then attach easily.

If, however, it is found out with this test that the retina is still totally or partly immobile, the cause should be looked for. It is recommendable to look for causes of the immobility in this succession: first to look for epiretinal membranes and vitreous remnants, then subretinal proliferations and as last the possible contraction of the retina itself. Most frequently it is tangential traction by the remaining membranes or vitreous remnants. They should then be removed in the described way. The subretinal proliferations are, after cleaning of the retina surface, visible through the retina, but they are not necessarily relevant for immobility of the retina. With two blunt instruments it is mostly easy to find out whether the retina is elevated by subretinal strands. Pressing on two points far from one another, one tries to press the retina against the pigment epithelium. With this manipulation it is very easy to see whether a counter-effect is coming from subretinal proliferations.

However, in the idiopathic detachments with PVR subretinal proliferations are, exceptionally, the additional cause of detachment. They occur much more frequently in traumatic cases and therefore the technique of their removal will be described there in detail. Subretinal proliferations, frequently in shape of strands which are sometimes to be seen with long existing detachments in myopic eyes and play no mechanical part in the detachment, should be left alone.

The last cause of immobility of the retina should be sought in the retina itself. The histopathologic basis of this change, in our opinion, has never been clearly described in connection with clinical situation, and we shall neglect it in the description of the situation and its surgical solution. It probably has to do with secondary changes of the retinal parenchym as consequence of the proliferative process and long-existing retinal detachment.

Simplifying a little, it could be said that, mainly, there are two different, clinically relevant situations. The first is when after removal of membranes the retina stays immobile and stiff. Frequently it looks as if the retina were a cast of the removed membranes (very marked with long-existing local diabetic traction detachments). Sometimes the whole retina is engaged, but much more frequently this change is local and corresponds to the most marked fixed retinal folds before removal of the membranes. It is also very frequent with long-existing detachments. Such an immobile retina in combination with peripheral tears cannot, or only with great difficulty, become attached through the silicone injection. When in such cases with silicone injecting the limit of the retina elasticity is reached, the surface tension of the silicone bubble will 'break' and silicone will come behind the retina through the tear. If there are no tears, the possibility to attach the retina is much greater, but there is also a considerable risk to tear the retina when the elasticity limit is reached. Thus it is best to mobilize the retina before silicone is injected at all.

Mechanical unfolding and mobilizing of the retina with two instruments is one of the possibilities, but it is rather risky. When pulling at the retina it can very easily tear. A better and less dangerous manipulation is the 'massage' of the retina with a blunt instrument. With the contracted retina this is achieved best if a 'massage' is applied to the retina with the back of the membrane peeler or if the retina is very gently sucked with the back flush needle with silicone brush and unfolded and flattened from the centre to the periphery. After 5–10 min it can be noticed that the folds are less rigid and the retina more mobile. In such a situation the retina is more contracted than shortened through long and forced immobility. After the mobilization a nearly complete reattachment of the retina is achieved with the silicone injection. Some remaining folds will disappear by themselves in a few days after surgery. A 'relaxing retinotomy' is in such situations mostly not necessary and sometimes, when introduced too early, even contraproductive and harmful.

The second situation is to be found in very old cases of retinal detachment with PVR. The proliferative process seems to be 'burnt-out' and the retina is very thin and transparent. After removal of the membranes it is conspicuous that the retina is not much folded, sometimes it is even smooth, but the vessels are very close together. The retina is very tense and it is difficult to open the funnel to the disc. One gets the impression that the retinal parenchym has partly disappeared (no folds, vessels close together). The retina is shortened and tears very easily. If the shortening is only radial (no funnel, the central retina around the disc can provisionally be flattened with two instruments without difficulty, without building concentric folds around the disc) then it is best to perform a circular retinotomy of at least 180° far peripherally. A further extension of the retinotomy can be done later if the retina still appears under traction, until the complete release is achieved.

The case is much more difficult if besides the radial shortening also a circular shortening is present. In this situation after removal of the membranes the retina looks like a mushroom in which the central retina, shrunk in the shape of a narrow funnel, represents the stem of the mushroom. The tendency that always emerges with the view on this situation, namely to perform a large radial retinotomy has to be suppressed immediately. The cutting of the retina radially from the periphery to the centre has to go up to the disc if contraction will be eliminated. After the cut the contracted retina will shrink and a large part of the pigment epithelium will remain uncovered. The remaining circular contraction of the central retina will still exist further in the shape of a half circular fold close to the disc. Flattening of the central retina after that is impossible.

The circular contraction is best to be treated before peripheral retinotomy is performed. As long as the retina is not separated from the periphery it can be tried to release circular contraction and further to widen the funnel with blunt instruments and best with both hands. It has to occur very carefully and takes rather much time, because rough and impatient manipulating can easily cause haemorrhage and retinal tears. This manipulation is continued until the disc is completely free and only a flat concentric retinal fold has remained of the funnel. After that radial shortening can be removed by means of retinotomy as

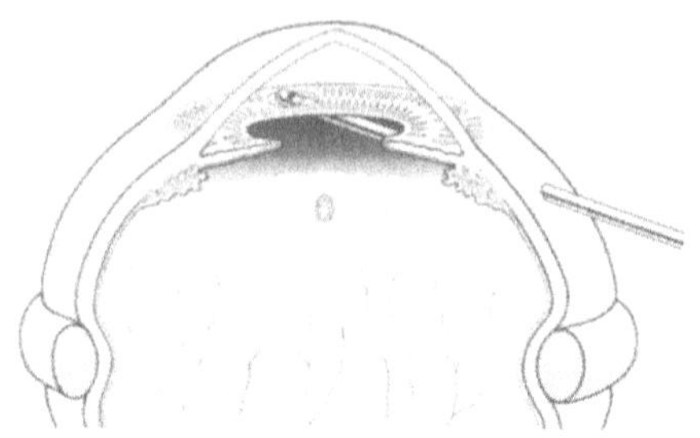

Figure 8. Six o'clock iridectomy.

described above. Even in the favourable cases a circular fold will continue to exist after the silicone injection. It will, though, disappear spontaneously in a short time after surgery. The described manipulation can only be performed within limits. In a strongly contracted retina, in which the funnel is very narrow and more than 2–3 mm deep, this manipulation will unfortunately be unsuccessful.

After vitrectomy with membranectomy and mobilization of the retina, the retina should be fixed definitely with the silicone injection. Before the silicone is injected the 6 o'clock iridectomy should be made first. The role of the iridectomy is to create a connection between the posterior and the anterior chamber, and to ensure that the produced aqueous enters the anterior chamber and so keeps the silicone bubble off the cornea. The function of iridectomy and complications with failing of the function will be described in detail in the description of the postoperative course.

Iridectomy is performed best after vitrectomy. Performance of iridectomy immediately after removal of the lens can have miosis as consequence, which then can make peripheral vitrectomy more difficult. Iridectomy is done best with the vitrectome. First the iris is sucked up from behind to detect the iris base (in very wide pupils sometimes difficult) and subsequently iridectomy is performed (Fig. 8). The iridectomy should better be big than small and every bleeding from the iris roots or the ciliary body should be stopped, because late bleeding and fibrin reaction in the area of iridectomy can close the hole in the postoperative course. The bleeding place can be controlled best with scleral depression. The area is so indented with cotton swab that the back surface of the iris and the ciliary processes are presented. With endodiathermy through sclerotomy the bleeding places are then coagulated.

It is advisable after iridectomy, before starting the silicone injection, to re-examine the fundus. Unexpected haemorrhages should be sought (especially if retinal surgery has been performed before). The intravitreal space, and also the subretinal space if large retinotomies are made, should be free from blood, pigment clumps and other debris as much as possible before silicone oil

56

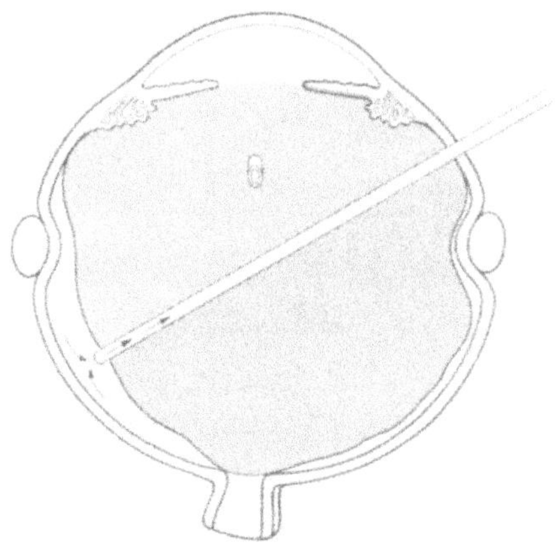

Figure 9. Endodrainage with adapted pressure of the silicone.

is injected. The same holds for the retina. Blood clots on or under the retina can, under circumstances, make unfolding and attachment of the retina under silicone oil considerably difficult.

Bulbus hypotony with exchange from fluid to silicone infusion is to a certain extent avoidable through closing of the sclerotomy opening with sclerotomy plugs. After that the infusion fluid tube on the infusion cannula is simply exchanged with the silicone oil tube. It is best to hold the cannula with a needle holder and to exchange the infusion tubes with the other hand. In this way unpleasant air bubbles in the silicone injection are avoided. Expansion of silicone oil can best be observed through the contact lens holding the endo-illumination in one hand and the back-flush needle in the other. The silicone injection can best be started with maximum pressure of the silicone oil pump, because the bulbus is still strongly hypotonic in the beginning.

Drainage of the fluid through the needle will only function when the inner pressure has passed the level of the outer pressure. In the not bullously detached retina the intravitreal fluid can be evacuated first. Only when silicone oil has reached the retina in the posterior pole, the retinal hole or retinotomy is sought and drainage of the subretinal fluid is started. There it is often sufficient to hold the opening of the needle in front of the retinal hole to initiate a fluid stream. Scraping on the pigment epithelium is to be avoided. The back flush needle with the silicone brush is particularly suitable for this manipulation, because it does not easily damage the retina and the pigment epithelium. The eye pressure has to be regulated with the silicone pump so that it is only slighty higher than the outer pressure, which is sufficient for a continuous stream of the fluid through the needle (Fig. 9). A too high pressure would 'dry out' the endodrainage place too fast and abruptly, and particularly if the place is peripheral, it would capture the remaining subretinal fluid

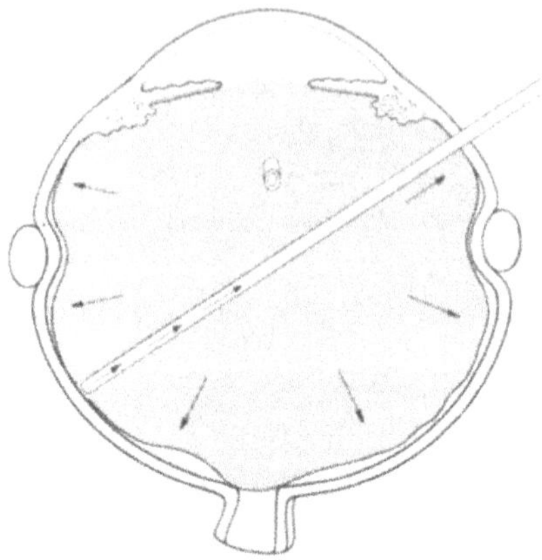

Figure 10. Endodrainage with too high pressure of the silicone – subretinal fluid is captured and not in contact with the back-flush needle any more.

central from the place (Fig. 10). In spite of lowering of the pressure sometimes it will not be possible to initiate the fluid stream again, and a new more central retinotomy will be necessary to evacuate the fluid.

In the bullous detachment silicone oil will reach the retina quickly and, if the intravitreal space is drained simultaneously, at a certain moment the detachment will optically increase. Because of the expansion of the silicone bubble on the retinal periphery, the peripheral subretinal fluid is pressed under the central retina and the bullous detachment will move from the periphery to the central part of the retina. In this situation the subretinal fluid has to be drained simultaneously with the silicone injection through the pre-existing central hole or through a performed retinotomy.

In this way in a very short time the retina is brought so far that it is unfolded and still flatly detached. To drain the remaining subretinal fluid completely takes a little longer and demands some patience and skilful manipulating with the eye pressure. In the end a very small volume is concerned, so that excessive rise of the pressure can be reached easily. In this phase observation of the vessels on the disc is a good standard for the regulation of pressure. Injecting of silicone oil is regulated with the pump pedal. However, the excessive increase of the pressure can frequently not be avoided. The fastest regulation of the increased pressure is the release of silicone oil through the sclerotomy. Therefore it is very important that both sclerotomies are free from vitreous and other tissue and that in every moment the silicone oil can be released by taking out one of the two instruments from the eye.

Drainage of the remaining subretinal fluid is also dependent on the mobility of the retina. In a completely unfolded mobile retina, where the subretinal space is not divided by folds into various small pockets, it is also easy to completely drain from the periphery. On the other hand, a somewhat contracted and folded retina cannot, even with several retinotomies and hard drainage attempts, become completely attached.

This should be kept in mind, and in a mobile retina one should not perform the central retinotomy unnecessarily, nor in a contracted retina try to drain the last drop of the fluid at the expense of many retinotomies. The complete drainage is very useful, if only that the optimal silicone oil filling can be reached in this way, but it is also something that has not to be reached absolutely and at any cost. Just as in the conventional surgery and in the rhegmatogenous detachments the pigment epithelium pump will take care of the resorption of the fluid and many a folded retina will become flat again and unfold through its own elasticity after some time. These forces may not be overvalued either, but it is very useful to think of them in the phase of the operation when one can advance only with dubious and aggressive manipulations.

The complete or nearly complete attachment of the retina is followed by the retinopexy as the last procedure. As we have used almost exclusively cryocoagulation with our patients, we shall describe it here. Laser coagulation, certainly central from the buckle, can also be used just as well, if not even better.

The endocryopexy is performed 360° peripherally from the buckle edge, continuously and in two or three rows. In the area where visibility is not satisfying the periphery is indented and coagulated centrally, the edges of the defects and retinotomies are supplied continuously with a row of coagulates. If a microcryo probe is not available, a common cataract probe can also be applied. The sclerotomy has then to be widened a little, the probe is mostly 1.3–1.5 thick, and the insulation tube should be removed from the probe. With the coagulation it should be kept in mind that the probe is not insulated and that the sclerotomy place can also be frozen. Waiting for a few seconds before the probe is moved to another place can prevent unpleasant bleedings from the sclerotomy site. Bleeding following cryocoagulation, caused by the developed hyperaemy (sometimes also mechanically), is frequently to be seen. Therefore it is very advisable to examine the coagulated area after coagulation of a quadrant. If a bleeding is discovered the coagulation should be interrupted and the bleeding stopped. The accumulated and coagulated blood under the silicone oil is sometimes difficult to remove and should therefore be avoided. After cryocoagulation the fundus should be examined. Nearly always it is possible to detect that some fluid coming from the periphery gathered again in front of the disc. It should be sucked out.

Before the sclerotomies are closed the anterior chamber should be checked. If the silicone oil has filled the whole anterior chamber, some fluid should be injected through the iridectomy. Before injection some silicone oil should be evacuated from the eye to decrease the pressure. In the soft eye the injected fluid will stay in the anterior chamber and push the silicone bubble backwards. In the hypertonic and normotonic eye this will not be possible and the whole amount of fluid that is injected will get behind the silicone bubble and in front of the disc, and it has to be evacuated again. To insist on the fluid pushing the silicone oil bubble completely behind the iris is not necessary. It is already sufficient if the fluid has cleared the iridectomy from silicone oil. In this way the produced aqueous will find the way and push the silicone bubble farther behind the diaphragm.

When closing the sclerotomy openings the attention should be paid to leaving the bulbus with a normal intraocular pressure. With a normal intraocular pressure no special positioning of the patient is necessary.

A high pressure, on the contrary, combined with the normal supine position of the patient after the surgery can, under circumstances, cause accumulation of the aqueous behind the silicone bubble and a pupillary block.

After closing of the sclerotomies and before closing of the conjunctiva the whole operating field is carefully washed out with saline to prevent the silicone oil from staying in the wound and appearing under the conjunctiva after the operation. It should be washed particularly well if the Tenon capsule was opened further backward (primary encircling procedure). No mydriatic drops are put in the eye to prevent the possible closing of the iridectomy. In very wide pupils a miotic ointment can be given to open the iridectomy.

Giant tears

As we have mentioned briefly at the indications, the degree of difficulty with a giant tear is much more determined by the degree of development of the proliferative process than by the size of the tear itself. The surgical technique is also adapted to this fact, and in the following section we shall describe the surgical technique in various situations. Although, obviously, pathological situations do not differ sharply and change gradually into one another, it still seems useful to divide them into several groups:
- recent giant tears without manifested PVR;
- giant tears with manifested PVR and a mobile retina; and
- giant tears with progressed PVR and an immobile retina.

With the first group, fresh giant tears, a small number of cases is not operated in this technique, as we have mentioned before. These are the recent tears in the upper area and without detachment, which can be operated successfully with air-gas injection, a buckle and mostly without vitrectomy.

The beginning of the operation with the greatest part of the group is the same as with other PVR cases. Placing of the encircling band and lensectomy are performed in the above described manner. As mostly young patients are concerned, lensectomy presents no difficulties. The retina is frequently inverted and lying on the bottom of the eye. As the retina is very mobile, it is best to let it lie there until vitrectomy has been finished. Vitrectomy behind the ciliary body and in the area of the vitreous base follows in the described manner, with scleral indentation. In the area of the tear it is practically impossible to remove the vitreous from the peripheral tear edge and it is not necessary either. It is best to remove the remaining retina together with the vitreous. Removal of the vitreous from the retina and sometimes from the central edge of the tear is a little more difficult and should, because of mobility of the retina, be performed with adjusted sucking power of the vitrectome. Only after a complete vitrectomy should the reposition of the inverted retina be performed. It is best to use the back-flush needle with silicone tip and suck the tear edge in the middle of the tear (Fig. 11). It is always a fascinating moment of the surgery when the disc appears again from behind the inverted retina. When the retina is completely free from the vitreous, with a fresh giant tear, it will fall back and almost reattach spontaneously and further manipulations are mostly superfluous. It should be noticed that it is useful to examine the exposed pigment epithelium. Sometimes pigment clumps can be found, especially around the disc. These should be sucked off with the back-flush needle without touching pigment epithelium. The same should be done with the surface of the retina after reposition. The pigment cells and clumps are frequently to be found in the lower region and frequently already slightly stuck to the retina. They also ought to be removed.

The silicone oil injection follows in the usual manner. As the retina mostly lies on the bottom almost completely unfolded, manipulating with the retina during the injection is not necessary. The entire activity may be limited to observation of the expansion of the silicone bubble and sucking off of the fluid with the back-flush needle. When the silicone bubble has reached the peripheral retina, one can start unfolding of the remaining retinal folds with the back-flush needle.

Under moderate intraocular pressure the retina is sucked up with the back-flush needle and then moved to the corresponding place in the periphery (Fig. 12). With the finger pressure on the silicone tube of the needle the retina is then pressed out and left in the place. The advantage of the back-flush needle is that the retina can be not only peripherally but also, if necessary, centrally, sucked up and moved. The necessary intraocular pressure is always regulated simultaneously with the foot pedal of the silicone pump. Alternately also the pre- and subretinal liquid is evacuated. Evacuation of the subretinal liquid occurs mostly without problems, because the retina is so mobile. Evacuation can also be performed through the tear itself and a central retinotomy is hardly ever needed. In this way, with a little patience and skill, even the largest giant

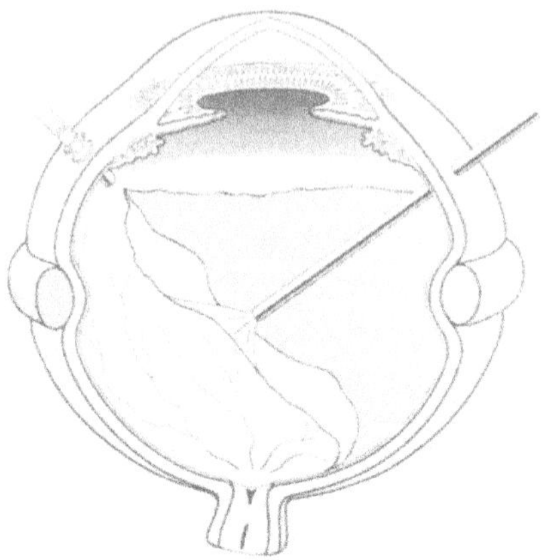

Figure 11. Repositioning of the retina with the flute needle.

tears of 270° and more can be treated. It should be noticed that with giant tears larger than 180° the retina is sometimes twisted, especially if it is completely mobile. This is best to be seen at the course of the vessels. With the reposition, this should be taken into account and the folded and twisted retina should be gradually moved peripherally in the direction opposite to the twisting. The final right position of the retina is again assessed after the course of the vessels. Slipping of the retina in the direction of the disc under the silicone, when the retina is completely unfolded and placed in the original position, is seldom observed. If at the end of the operation slipping is stated, it is the sign that the retina is not in the right position (twisting) or that too much subretinal fluid has remained before and behind the retina. Corresponding measures have then to be taken. At the end of the operation endocryopexy is performed. The tear edge is coagulated with one row of coagulates and the remaining retina with two rows, peripherally to the buckle.

Surgical technique with giant tears with manifested PVR and mobile or immobile retina will be described for both groups together. The assessment of mobility of the retina is not possible preoperatively and is only done during surgery. If after vitrectomy and removal of proliferative membranes the retina remains contracted and immobile, the operative procedure has to be expanded and further surgical measures such a retinotomy and retina fixation have to be applied.

The clinical picture of giant tear with PVR varies from case to case and depends, among other things, very much on the duration of existence of the tear. In all cases all characteristics of the PVR are there very early. Beside nearly always existing total detachment, the retina is almost totally immobile, particularly the torn half. It is covered with epiretinal membranes and tear edges are always curled and fixed. The other half of the retina can still be

62

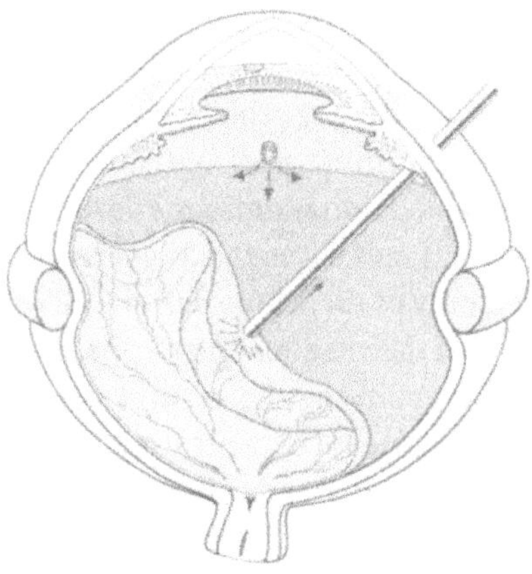

Figure 12. Unfolding of the retina under the silicone with the back-flush needle.

relatively smooth, but it is also covered with membranes. Subretinal proliferations, at least with fresh cases, are rare. The vitreous is completely contracted and, with older cases, also completely immobile. It can very well be seen at the peripheral tear edge and the peripheral edge of the torn retina. It is totally immobile and pulled forwards by sagital vitreous contraction. It is interesting to notice that with giant tears with progressed PVR an entirely inverted retina and covered disc occur in a much smaller number than with quite fresh giant tears. It is possible that the proliferative process with its contractive force partly pulls back and unfolds the inverted retina.

The described picture changes quickly and drastically after unsuccessful surgery in which no silicone oil was used. As the vitreous was removed during surgery, there is no counteracting force which can oppose tangential traction of epiretinal membranes. Therefore the retina is much more folded and contracted. The proliferative process has been stimulated by the preceding unsuccessful operation and progressed strongly. The pathoanatomic picture is dominated by two characteristic features: the peripheral retina (where it is not torn) is strongly adherent to the vitreous trunk, as vitrectomy in the base area mostly has not be performed radically, and epiretinal membranes are very massive and strongly adherent to the surface of the retina. This situation makes the re-operation of a giant tear with PVR technically much more difficult and prognostically much more unfavourable. This confirms our conviction that, certainly in these cases, silicone oil has to be used in the first operation.

Vitrectomy of the central vitreous is mostly without problems and occurs after lensectomy in the above described manner. Vitrectomy in the area of the vitreous base is combined with removal of the peripheral retina in the area of the giant tear. In these preoperated cases the vitreous remnants in the periphery are strongly adherent to the retina and frequently covered with membranes.

Vitreous remnants in the periphery can best be removed under coaxial light of the microscope with the vitrectome and scleral indentation. After that bimanual technique is applied and membranes are tried to be removed from the retina. In extremely difficult cases this is sometimes not possible and the only way out is a retinectomy of the whole peripheral retina so that a giant tear of 360° is made. Removal of the vitreous and peripheral membranes has mostly not much influence on mobility of the central retina, which is completely covered with membranes. Removal of central membranes begins from the disc to the periphery. In the torn half membranes are clearly visible and relatively easy to grasp. First an edge before the disc is sought with the short spatula, which is then changed for the forceps. Removal of membranes occurs relatively easily up to the curled edge of the torn retina. As they are there strongly adherent and very difficult to remove, one confines oneself first to cleaning the torn part of the retina up to the curled edges. The other half is frequently, especially in fresh cases, relatively smooth and there are no membranes visible on it. However, the surface of the retina is shiny with typical reflex and somewhat immobile on the whole. One should not be misled by the good appearance of the retina compared to the other half. Membranes are there and ought to be removed. It happened to us more than once in the past that after a few days or weeks we could observe reproliferations with subsequent re-detachments exactly from these places. For discovering and removing of these membranes the scratcher and the pick forceps are the most suitable instruments.

As most of the time a healthy and not atrophic retina is concerned, the scratcher can be used a little more aggressively without fear that the retina may be torn. This rather aggressive manoeuvre can locate membranes as well. The retina cleaned in this way will then be gently sucked with the back-flush needle and smoothed from the centre to the periphery. With this useful manoeuvre the last membrane remnants are removed from the surface of the retina and the contracted retina becomes more mobile. Soon afterwards it will be discovered that the torn half of the retina is much more immobile than the other one. A part of this immobility can be attributed to curled tear edges, where membranes have not been completely removed. It is also easy to notice optically that many radial folds have their origin in these peripheral contractions of the edge.

Experience has taught us that removal of membranes from tear edges and mobilizing of this part of the retina is a very arduous work, which often ends in an even more torn and still quite immobile retina. Therefore, for many years we have decided to amputate this part of functionally incapable retina. To prevent haemorrhage and to make removal of the avital retina easier the

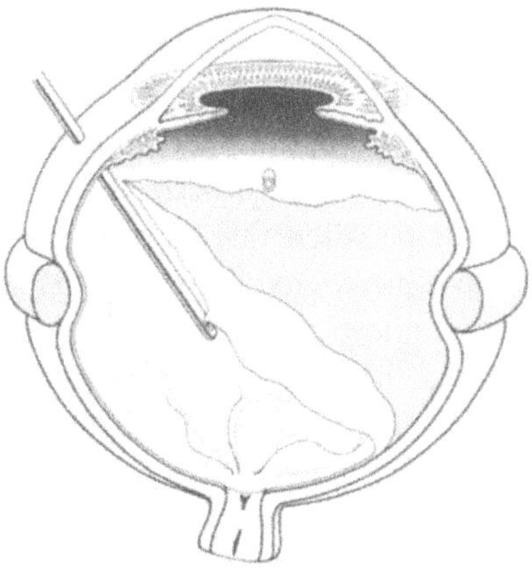

Figure 13. Removal of fibrotic and curled tear edges.

whole edge of the retina is coagulated with the endodiathermy probe. To remove the coagulated retina it is best to use the vitrectome with moderate sucking force. Sometimes the sucking alone is sufficient to remove the coagulated necrotic retina (Fig. 13). Remaining free necrotic parts of the coagulated edge can best be removed with back-flush needle. The retina can then be unfolded. If secondary haemorrhage from the vessels on the edge occurs, they have to be coagulated again.

After the removal of curled and immobile edges of the tear it will be noticed immediately that the retina is much more mobile and shows the tendency to attach. Subsequently the subretinal space and the back surface of the retina ought to be checked. On the back surface, particularly in the periphery, pigment clumps and onsets of proliferative membranes can sometimes be found. They should be removed with the back-flush needle or the forceps. Their removal only promotes mobility of the retina.

Before starting silicone injection the behaviour of the retina should be examined. The infusion bottle is placed in the highest position and simultaneously one tries to drain the subretinal space. Although the communication between the intravitreal and subretinal space is very large owing to the great tear, a mobile retina will show the tendency to attach through the strong pressure of the infusion fluid.

Silicone injection follows in the described way and differs from the already described procedure perhaps only in so far as the torn half of the retina has to be held with an instrument (back-flush needle or light pipe) during silicone expansion until silicone has reached the retina. After that the complete attachment of the retina with silicone injection and simultaneous evacuation of the fluid is, actually, achieved even faster than with quite fresh giant tears. This occurs because after removal of the epiretinal membranes this retina is still rather stiff and immobile compared to the retina with quite fresh giant tears. This retina folds much less and follows the pressure of the expanding silicone bubble much more flexibly and attaches much faster without many folds. Evacuation of the remaining fluid and endocryopexy at the end of the operation are performed in the above described way.

Another situation develops when the retina remains immobile after the vitrectomy. This situation is mostly to be found with long-existing giant tears, where the retina has been under the membranes for a long time and after removal of the membranes shows no tendency whatsoever to unfold. This retina has completely lost its elasticity and floats totally immobile as a cast of the membranes that have just been removed. As this retina is completely separated from the periphery in its whole length by the tear, it is not possible to attach it with silicone injection. Yet if one nevertheless tries one will find out immediately that, because the retina is not flexible, silicone soon reaches behind the retina. Therefore this retina should first become loose and mobile. This may be attempted in the following way. With the back-flush needle with a silicone tip one tries to suck it up lightly and sucking by 'massage' it from the centre to the periphery. With apropriate intraocular pressure it is an atraumatic treatment that can be repeated several times. After some time it will slowly become clear that the retina can unfold and become mobile. Extension of the retina with two back-flush needles at two distant points is sometimes very helpful. After 10–15 min the desired effect will mostly be achieved and the retina will be so mobile as to be attached by silicone injection.

In a small number of cases this will not succeed completely and the retina will stay partly immobile. Sometimes (very seldom) the retina is not only contracted and immobile but also damaged (central holes) so that the described manoeuvres are not possible or permissible. In these cases the retina should be mechanically fixed before silicone injection. Inspired by the Japanese authors in 1980 we first tried transvitreal retina fixation with the retinal suture with these difficult cases. The suture technique is not new and it is copied from the sewing-machine technique. A thin hollow needle is supplied with a 5×0 suturamid thread and inserted through the pars plana incision. Under microscope control the retina and the bulbus wall are perforated in succession at the corresponding place. On the outer side the needle point is sought, the thread pulled through it and the needle retracted. This manoeuvre is repeated with about 3 mm distance. Hereby the needle point with the present thread loop is again sought from the outside and tightened. The free end of the thread (after the first stitch) is pulled through the loop and the needle retracted again. In this way it is possible, from the place of sclerotomy, to sew continuously an area of about 160°. At the end of the suture both ends of the thread are knotted on the sclera.

This fixation technique, although difficult, proved its worth and was used by us for a few years. Disadvantages of the technique were much more on the technical side, which made it very time-consuming, than concerning its reliability, which was satisfactory. Particularly with sewing far posterior, the continuous change from the inner to the outer side of the eye took much time. The continuous leakage of the fluid along the stitch point made seeking the needle point on the outer side difficult and complicated.

Therefore in 1983 we changed enthusiastically to the fixation technique with tacks, as it was introduced by Ando. This technique, in which the retina is fixed with plastic tacks, was much simpler and regarded as a permanent fixation of the retina in combination with silicone oil.

As, in our opinion, the retina does not need further fixation after complete attachment and silicone injection, we modified the technique in 1983 and introduced simple steel tacks with a suitable forceps. The instrument is described fully in the corresponding chapter.

The surgical procedure is very simple, in any case much simpler than the preparation that has to precede it.

Before inserting the closed forceps with the steel tack into the sclerotomy opening, one should determine the place where the retina will be fixed. This is done best with two instruments, by which the half of the retina is spread over the chorioid. In this way an overall view is achieved and the corresponding places on the retina and on the pigment epithelium can be noticed. Excessive precision is here superfluous, because the retina can compensate small deviations by its elasticity. Putting of the tack in the bulbus wall is much more simple and precise when the inner eye pressure is a little increased. Therefore the second sclerotomy opening has to be properly closed (with instruments or a sclerotomy plug). For the same reason the infusion should also be set in the highest position. Placing of the tack is done with the forceps from one of the two sclerotomy openings depending on the situation (Fig. 14). Penetrating of the bulbus wall requires certain strength and can always be felt well by hand. The bulbus wall will always be completely penetrated to avoid later falling out or down of the tacks. Retracting of the closed forceps presents no problems. After each tack it should be ascertained by optical control that the retina lies firmly fixed and at the same time the spot for the following tack should be determined. The retina should be fixed only on a few critical spots and it is completely superfluous to supply the whole retina edge with tacks. In two quandrants in which the retina is torn 180° three or four tacks suffice. After fixation of the retina it is advisable to ascertain that the retina is not too tense. It occurs sometimes, mostly in radial direction, when the retina is fixed with the tacks too peripherally. Moving of the tacks is easy to carry out and if necessary, should not be refrained from.

Silicone oil injection and simultaneous evacuation of the fluid follows in the familiar way. Cryopexy is also performed as described, the fixed retinal edge is

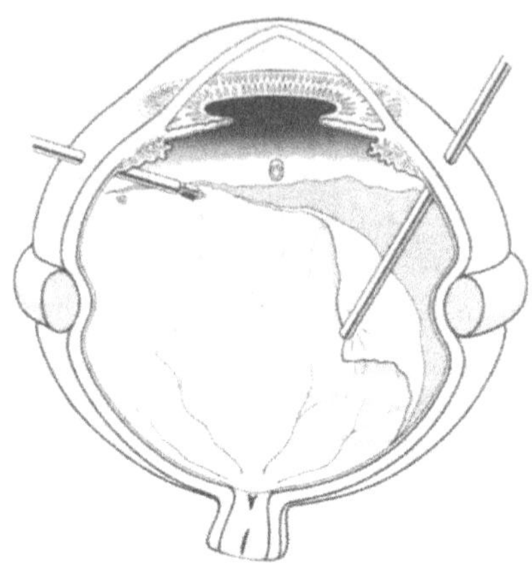

Figure 14. Transvitreal fixation with retinal tacks.

coagulated with a row of coagulates among the tacks, which are no obstacle for coagulation. At the end of the operation the tacks ought to be removed. After checking that all tackheads are sufficiently visible, the tacks are taken out one by one with the forceps (Fig. 15). To make the taking out easier and to prevent the occasional haemorrhage that might occur (very seldom), the inner eye pressure should be increased. Perforation sites do not need any further treatment after removal of the tacks and are not to be recognized shortly afterwards. A haemorrhage during the removing is as mentioned, extremely rare. We have never seen a haemorrhage from the perforation sites after the operation. If a haemorrhage occurs, it is easy to treat with increasing of the inner pressure and with endodiathermy.

At the end of this section a comment on retina fixation seems appropriate. Fixation of the retina with tacks is definitely an excellent technique, which is very simple and relatively without complications. By this and by certain radiation of magic it has lately become very popular. But just because of its simplicity it should be warned against its application when unnecessary and, which is even more important, at a too early stage of the operation. Permanent fixation of the retina has, understandably, no influence whatsoever on the course of the proliferative process, perhaps it even represents an additional, though small, provocation of proliferation. It can hardly be imagined that in case of a reproliferation the tacks could prevent traction detachment. Thus in our view, tacks should only be used as an instrument during surgery and removed after having served their purpose.

The tacks left in the eye after the operation mean, in many respects, a potential danger and a source of complications. As this difficult surgery, unfortunately, abounds in unavoidable complications, it does not seem necessary to introduce yet additional and avoidable ones.

68

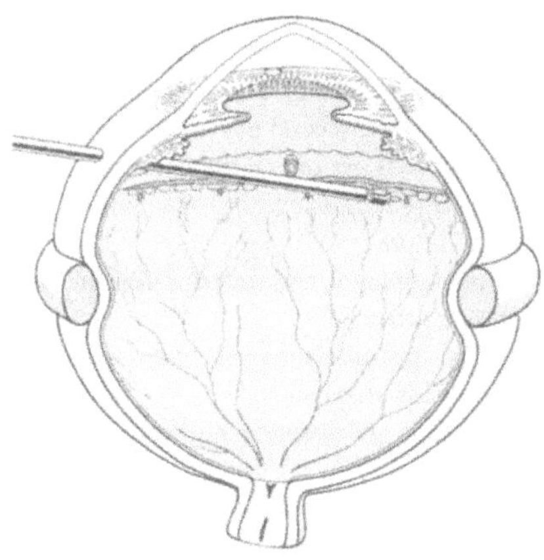

Figure 15. Removal of tacks after the silicone injection.

Besides the question in which way tacks should be used, the questions in which stage of the operation and how frequently they should be used are at least equally important. The simplicity with which tacks can be set is very tempting and the tendency to place them at the early stage of the operation, when the retina is not yet completely clean and mobile, is very evident. Such retina, forced and fixed with tacks may look quite good at the end of the operation, but the joy will, unfortunately, be brief and reproliferation with succeeding redetachment from not removed membranes will occur in a short time. If during the operation one opposes this tendency – to use tacks too soon – and tries to clean the retina from membranes and mobilize it in all by now described ways, one will discover after some time that tacks are not so often necessary at all. Perhaps it is a good advice not to have sterile and ready-to-use tacks on the instrument table at all, but have them sterilized every time before using. This threshold will frequently suffice to mobilize the retina further and to abstain from setting the tacks.

In conclusion it could be said that tacks for fixation of the retina, as well as other surgical techniques in the retinal surgery, should be used only after much consideration and as the last remedy.

Traction detachment with PVR after perforating trauma

Traction detachments with PVR developed after perforating injuries are characterized by particular aggressivity of the proliferative process and by great tendency to re-proliferations. The proliferative process develops mostly in two ways. The first is growing of fibrotic tissue from the perforation scar. This process can be understood as an inadequate course of the normal scarring

Plate 1. Detachment with PVR operated after original Scott's technique.

1. Iatrogenic retinal tear made during an operation. It was possible to finish the operation successfully. Laser coagulation on the second day after the operation.
2. Due to postoperative contraction of peripheral membranes on the 5th day after an initially successful operation a tear occurred (or an existing one opened). Consequence: total detachment with silicone behind the retina.
3. Postoperative contraction of peripheral and anterior fibrotic structures after a successful operation – the central retina is attached.
4. Postoperative contraction of peripheral membranes with residual detachment after a successful operation – the central retina is attached.
5. Reproliferation of the membranes not dissected during the operation – the central retina is attached.
6. After the partly successful operation. A small silicone bubble is captured in residual peripheral membranes. Inferior redetachment.

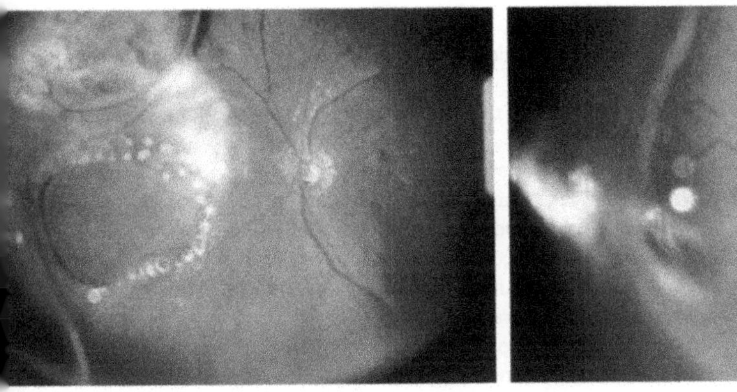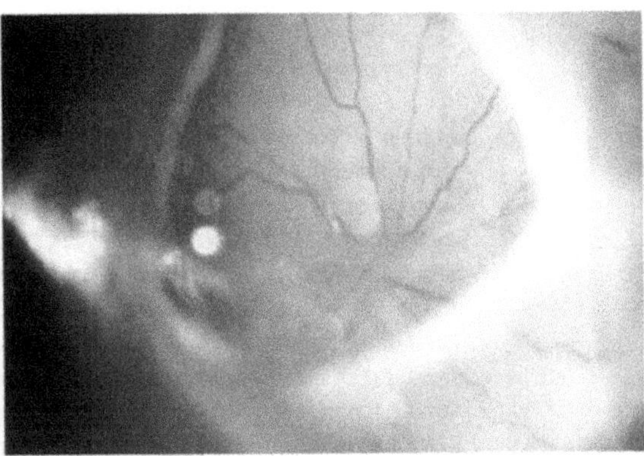

2

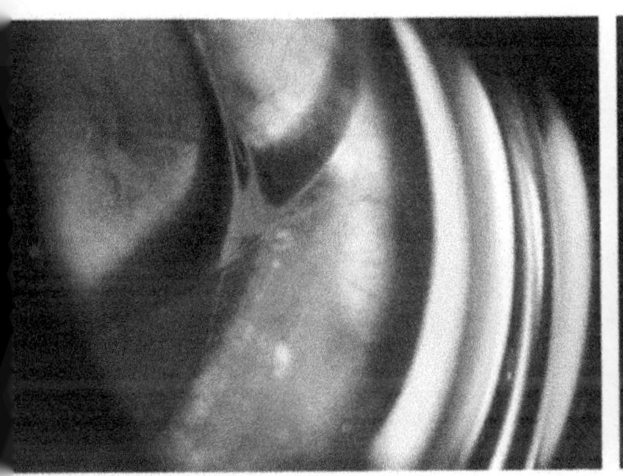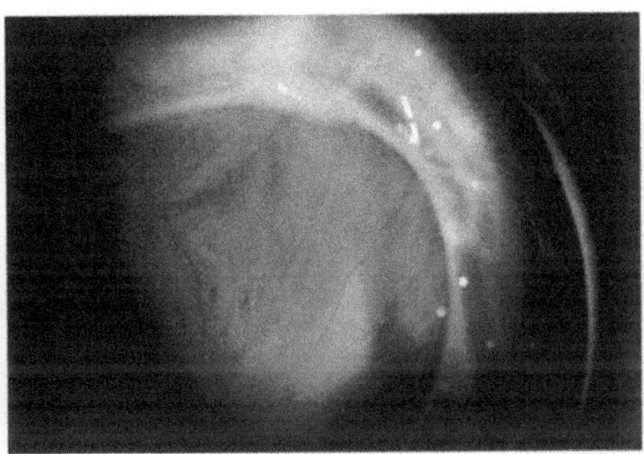

4

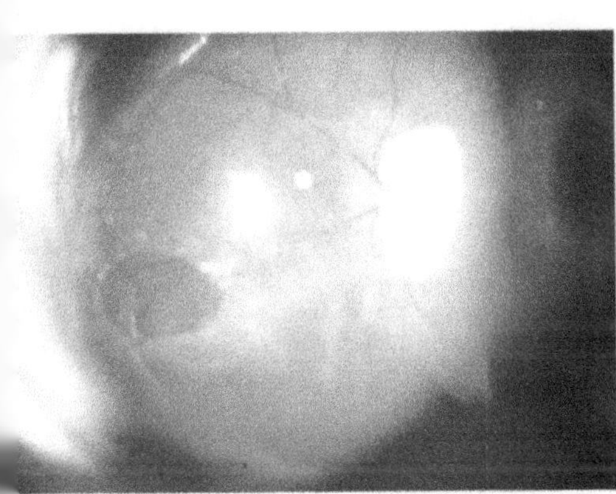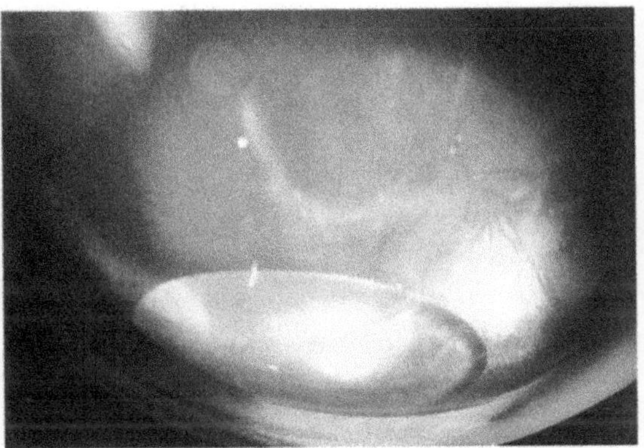

71

6

1. Very impressive picture of central proliferation with the closed funnel. Periphery is relatively free.
2. Situation after the operation. Ripe central membranes were relatively easy to remove. No retinal surgery.
3. Subtotal detachment, changes are concentrated in the periphery, the vitreous base reaching far posteriorly. Congenital high myopy (bilateral situation).
4. Situation after the operation: vitrectomy/lensectomy. Because of adherent membranes a nearly 360° retinectomy was necessary. Silicone tamponade.
5. Total detachment with PVR after unsuccessful conventional surgery. Closed funnel. Massive proliferative changes centrally and peripherally.
6. Total detachment with massive subretinal proliferation. Giant tear in a congenital myopy. Reproliferation after initially successful vitrectomy with the retina incarceration.

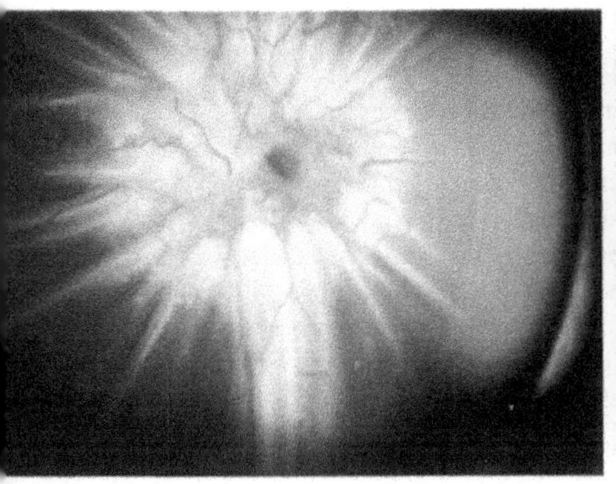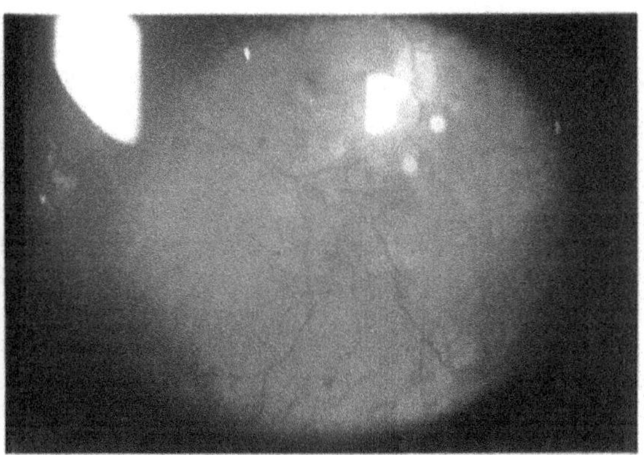

2

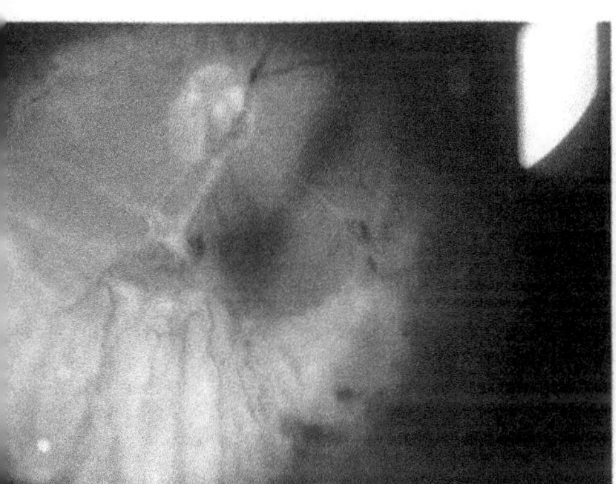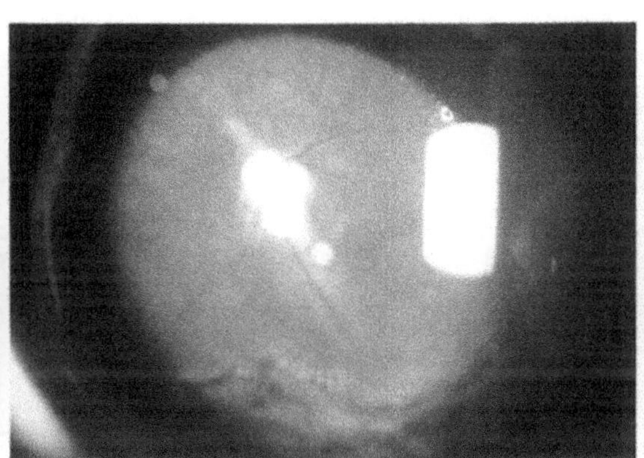

4

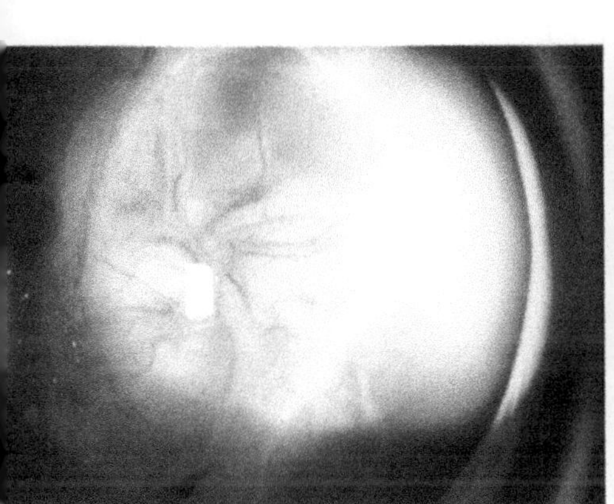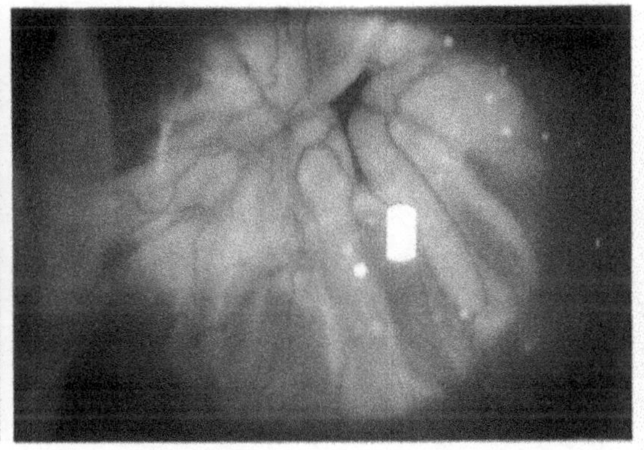

6

Plate 3. Giant tears.

1. Fresh giant tear of 270° with beginning PVR.
2. Situation after the operation: vitrectomy/lensectomy, silicone tamponade.
3. Giant tear of 180° of the nasal retina with manifested PVR.
4. Situation after the operation: after vitrectomy/lensectomy and silicone tamponade. Re-proliferation in the initially not involved temporal part of the retina.
5. Situation after the second operation: membrane peeling behind the silicone.
6. Traumatic giant tear after severe perforation. Situation after the operation: vitrectomy, partial retinotomy, peripheral silicone tamponade. Due to parapapillar contraction of the retina and incomplete retinotomy the macular area is moved to 12 o'clock position. Nevertheless, relatively good central vision 0,1 and central visual field.

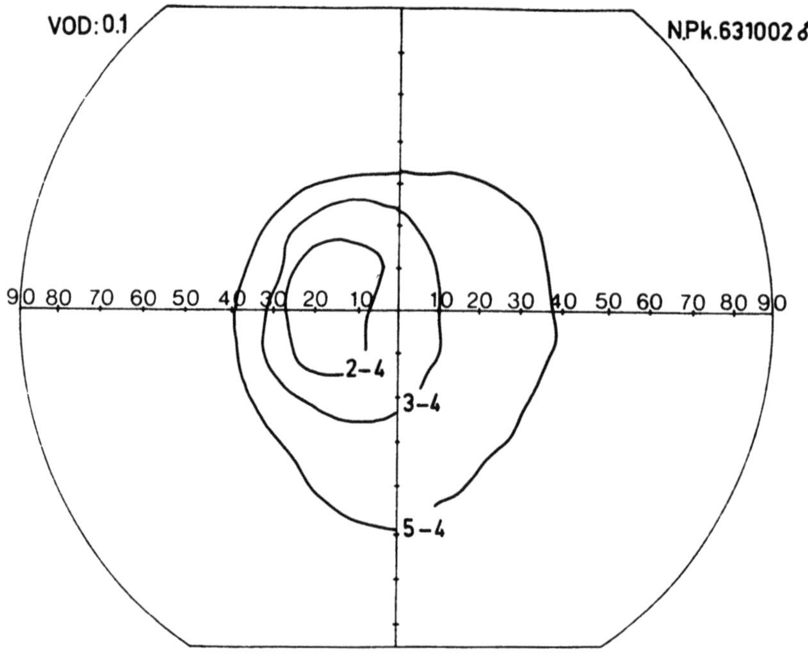

Visual field belonging to plate 3.6.

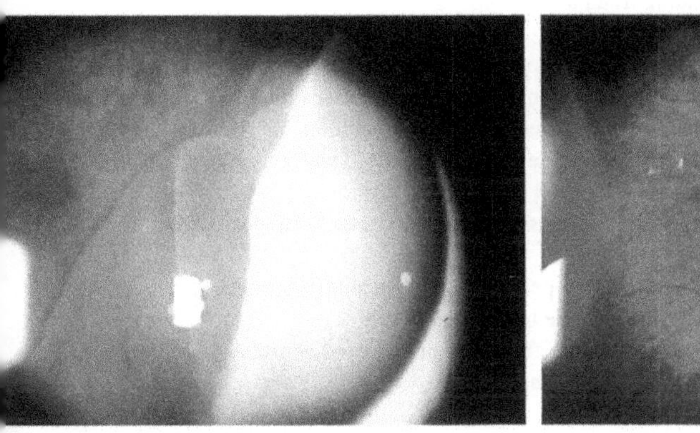
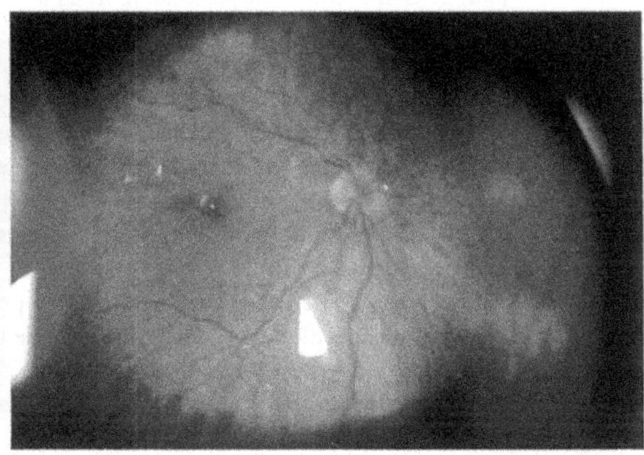

2

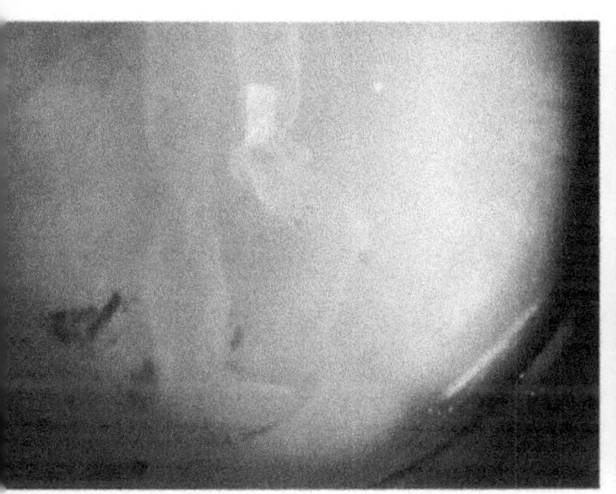
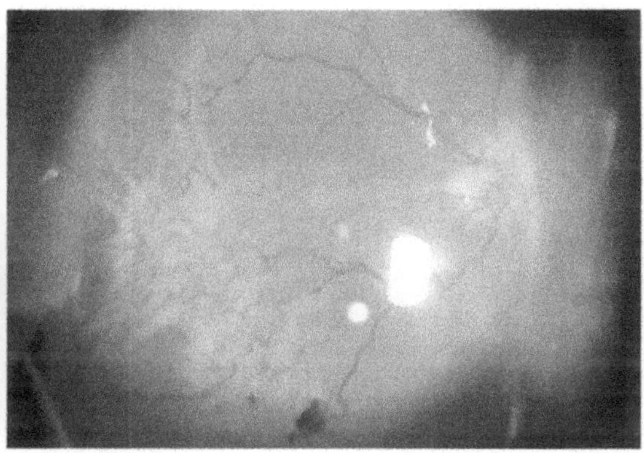

4

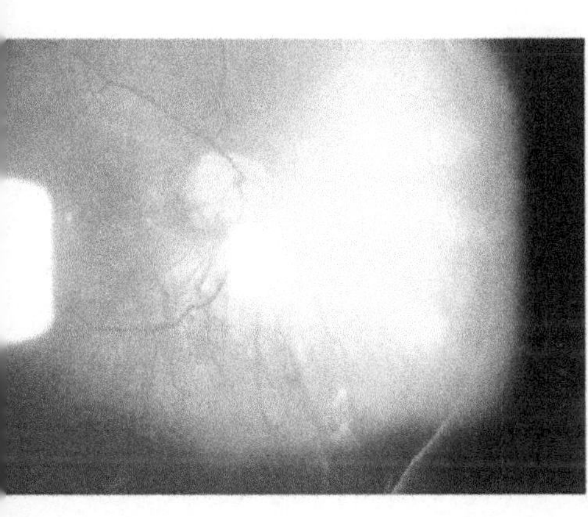
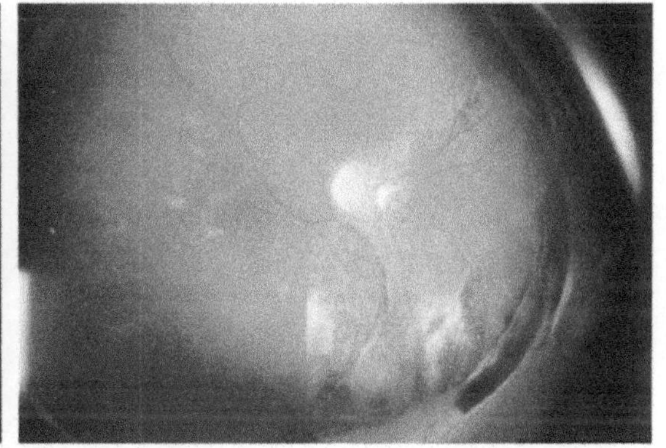

6

Plate 4. Giant tears after perforating trauma.

1. Giant tear of 340° with the incarcerated retina after a blunt trauma and bulbus rupture.
2. Situation after the operation: vitrectomy/lensectomy, 360° retinal suture with silicone tamponade – huge chorioidal detachment – 3 weeks after the operation.
3. Traumatic giant tear after vitrectomy and Healon tamponade. Totally contracted retina with manifested PVR.
4. Situation after the operation: vitrectomy/lensectomy, transvitreal fixation with tacks, silicone tamponade.
5. Traumatic giant tear – situation after four operations and a silicone injection. Massive epi- and subretinal proliferation, open tear, silicone behind the retina.
6. Situation after the operation: vitrectomy, removal of epi- and subretinal proliferations, retinectomy of the inferior retina, silicone tamponade.

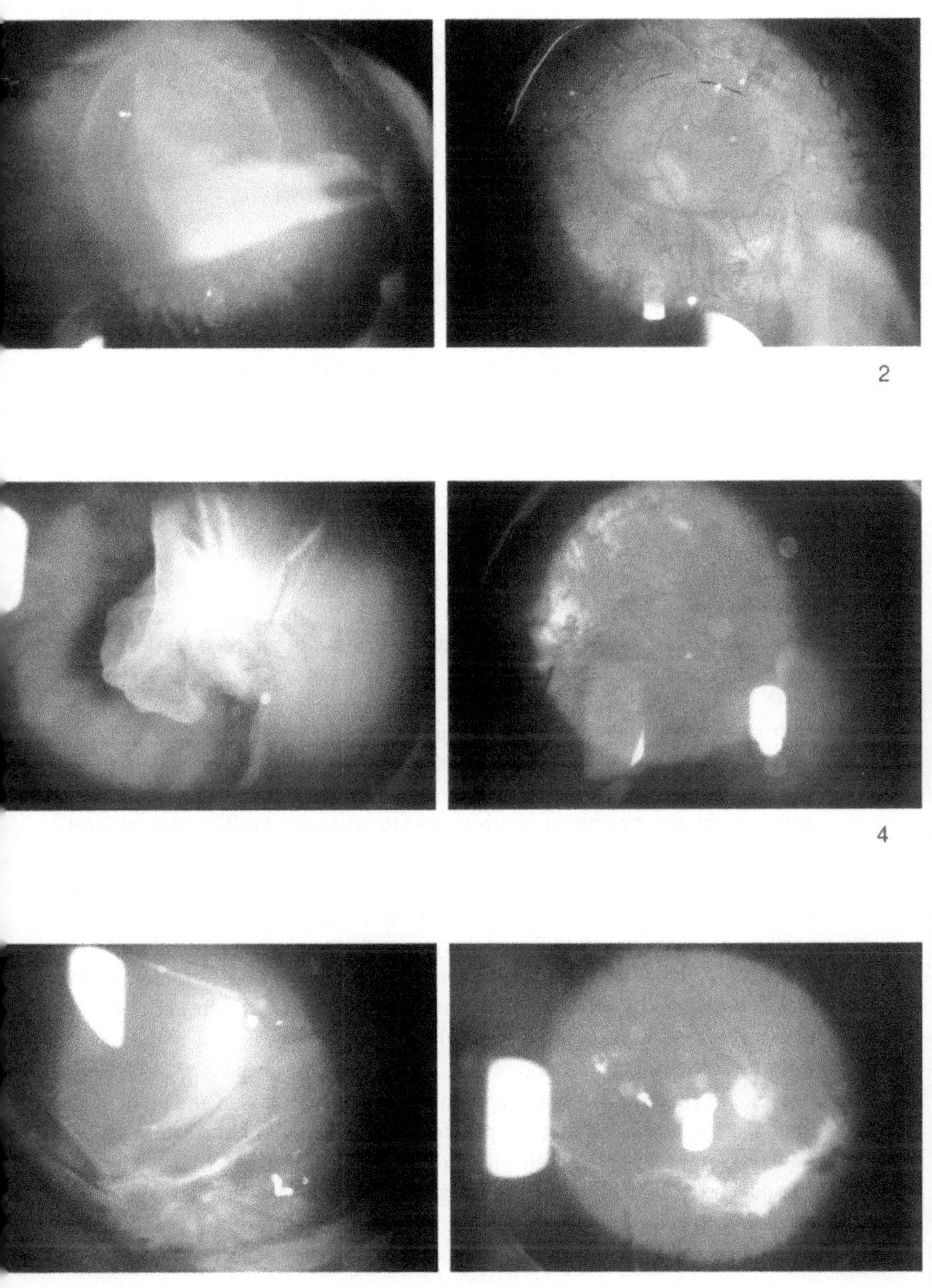

2
4
77
6

process. The second way is the cellular proliferation of the sedimented pigment cells on the free surface of the retina and the vitreous. The factors stimulating both processes are manifold and because of their importance worth enumerating:

1. perforating trauma frequently combined with contusion effect;
2. traction detachment developed by the trauma itself or later by the normal scarring process;
3. inflammatory reaction developed by presence of blood and lens-vitreous mixture in the eye;
4. hypotony developed by the traumatic shock by the direct injury of the ciliary body or by the secondary traction on the ciliary body;
5. rhegmatogenous factor – primary retinal tears developed at the time of the injury (less frequent) or secondary, developed by traction.

The combination of these factors leads to development of proliferative processes, which clinically manifest themselves mainly through three different mechanisms:

1. direct traction on the retina from the perforation scar combined with vitreous traction;
2. tangential traction of epiretinal membranes;
3. traction of subretinal proliferations mostly in the form of subretinal strands.

A number of typical pathoanatomic situations develops based on these mechanisms, which are, obviously, often combined with one another. In the following paragraphs we shall describe the surgical technique for particular situations.

Primary retinal detachment developed at the time of trauma occurs mostly with big sclerocorneal or corneal injuries with the loss of vitreous, lens or iris (Fig. 16). The cause is purely mechanical due to vitreous traction on the retina and has, in the beginning, nothing to do with the proliferative process. However, in such a pathoanatomic situation all stimulating factors as conditions for development of a PVR are present in a high degree, so that this situation can easily be regarded as the first step of PVR. Detachment is sometimes discovered with the primary wound repair, but mostly it is found at ultrasonic examination after a few days. The view into the posterior segment is mostly obstructed by presence of blood in the anterior part of the eye. The best time for the operation is at the end of the first or at the beginning of the second week after the primary wound repair. At this time the chances of a peroperative haemorrhage and of bursting of the wound are decreased and at the same time one can also hope that the proliferative process has not started yet.

The operation begins with placing of the encircling band. It is strongly recommended to examine the perforation wound closely at this stage and if necessary to reinforce it with a few stitches. While inserting the infusion it should be kept in mind that because of bad view, strong hypotony and possible

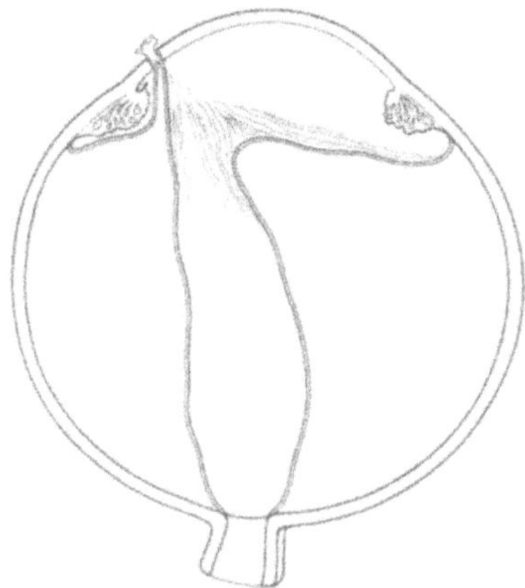

Figure 16. Incarceration of the vitreous with primary retinal detachment after the perforating trauma and the loss of the lens and the iris.

chorioidal haemorrhage, the infusion cannula can very easily stay behind the chorioid or behind the retina. An extra long 7 mm infusion cannula is to be preferred. In extremely hypotonic eyes, which are no rarity, it is much better first to insert the infusion with the long cannula and let the infusion flow to normalize the intraocular pressure, and then to tie the already placed encircling band. Too strong tightening of the encircling band is thus avoided.

Vitrectomy is started without the contact glass, in the anterior segment, with clearing away the blood. Caution is the top priority, because the retina is frequently pulled quite forwards, and when cleared from blood it is very mobile. The lens is often completely absent or the lens remnants are mixed with blood and vitreous. It is best to start vitrectomy in the middle, as it can be assumed that there the distance between the retina and the vitreous is greatest. When the retina has been discovered, it is best to work from the centre to the periphery and to use the retina as the orientation layer. Because of the detached vitreous this work is relatively easy until the vitreous base is reached. Separating of the opaque vitreous in the area of the vitreous base from the retina will be more difficult. It is best to leave the retina for the moment and try to clear away the lens remnants and blood by indenting the sclera in the area of the ciliary body. When the ciliary body is completely free, one starts the vitrectomy of the vitreous base. One tries, now working from the periphery to the centre, to clean the peripheral retina and in this way to meet the central retina, which has already been cleaned.

It is best to leave the area of the perforation scar as the last. The area of the perforation scar and the surrounding retina, which is sometimes incarcerated there, should be cleaned from blood and vitreous very thoroughly. With all these manoeuvres the opening of the vitrectome should never be held against the retina. It is best to hold the opening at the angle of 90° to the retinal surface. In this way the vitreous can be cut from the retina rather short without making holes. The described work is made very difficult by the bullous detached and mobile retina. In ideal situations it is possible to finish vitrectomy completely and so to assess the situation of the retina in relation to the perforation scar. However, very often this is not possible because the detached retina is in the way. In this situation it is recommendable to perform peripheral retinotomy and to drain the subretinal fluid. After that the mobile retina will, at least partly, attach and further working in the periphery will be possible. Simultaneously the assessment of the situation of the retina in relation to the perforation scar is much easier and more realistic with the less detached retina. In these cases the retina can be in contact with the perforation scar in many different ways. The first possibility is that the surrounding retina is incarcerated in the scar or sticks to the scar through blood and vitreous traction. It is basically mobile and folded only through the fixation with the scar. At this stage the proliferative process is not yet obvious, but the first onsets are already to be found. Therefore, in these badly damaged eyes, in which the proliferative process almost certainly exists and is particularly aggressive, there is no place for optimism in relation to the final result nor for any defensive surgery. As the retina is still mobile, in some cases it will be possible to free the retina from the scar without cutting it and to attach it without using silicone. However, the later traction, developed through contraction of the perforation scar and subsequently through the proliferative process, will pull the attached retina and very probably cause re-detachment. Therefore the surrounding retina has, in these cases, first to be completely cleaned from the vitreous and then separated from the scar. The fibrotic tissue of the scar should first be cut as short as possible. The surrounding retina, clean from blood and vitreous, should be coagulated around the scar with the diathermy probe and then separated from the scar stalk. To avoid secondary haemorrhage from the scar and to promote shrinking of the scar, the scar should be diathermocoagulated. The retina cut in this way will be later attached by means of silicone and coagulated.

A different situation is to be found particularly in large limbus-parallel scleral or corneal perforations with substantial loss of the vitreous. The opposite retina is incarcerated in the wound or pulled into the wound through vitreous incarceration. It always concerns the area of the vitreous base of the opposite retina. If the retina itself is incarcerated in the wound, there is no other way but to cut it out of the wound and so as it were to produce a giant tear. The surrounding retina will then be separated from the scar as described above. In this way after separating the retina from the scar there are two large retinotomies opposite to one another. The retina is very mobile and easily tears further. One should try in any case to leave a bridge of the retina on both

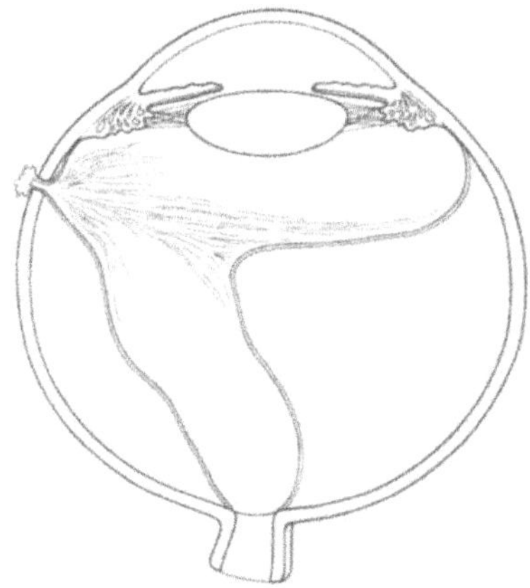

Figure 17. Incarceration of the retina after the perforating trauma.

sides between the two retinotomies. Attachment of the retina with silicone injection is thus made much easier.

If the opposite retina is only pulled to the scar by vitreous traction, retinotomy or retinectomy is not necessary (Fig. 17). It will be sufficient only to remove the vitreous so as to free the retina.

In all these manners the retina, cleaned from the vitreous and freed from the perforation scar, is mostly quite mobile and can be attached with silicone injection without much trouble, as it has been described with giant tears.

While injecting silicone one should not forget the relatively freshly repaired perforation wound. The wound should permanently be checked during the injection, and silicone should be injected with much caution regarding the intraocular pressure.

Another group is the secondary traction detachment with PVR developed some time after the perforating injury. These are mostly the eyes which are less damaged and recover functionally and anatomically after some time. After the acute loss of vision after the perforation the stage of subjective and objective recovery follows after a few weeks. The vitreous cleans up, the retina is attached and improvement of vision follows. This encouraging situation is unfortunately much too often the reason for the patient to evade control and for the surgeon to abandon precise control of the retinal periphery or the surroundings of the perforation scar. After some time, however, a traction detachment develops due to contraction of the perforation scar. A part of these cases, if operated in time, will be cured with conventional surgery. In the other part the proliferative process develops either spontaneously after some time or after the unsuccessful conventional operation. The time span of development after the trauma is not limited and can take from a few months to a few years.

A number of pathoanatomic situations develops through different kinds of injuries. Because of their specificity these situations demand corresponding specific surgical treatment and they should also be described separately.

Traction detachment with the centre in the periphery develops mostly after double perforation, foreign bodies or limbus parallel lacerations in the area of the ciliary body or anterior to the ora serratta. Detachment develops through direct traction of the contracting scar on the surrounding retina, or indirectly through vitreous traction on the opposite retina. Frequently a local cataract is found and the lens is often subluxated. With scars situated quite anteriorly there is often traction on the ciliary body, sometimes even detachment of the ciliary body. Very typical for scars lying between the ora and the ciliary body is a white fibrotic sheet spreading circularly on both sides of the scar. The retina is involved in various ways by traction starting from the scar. If no holes exist, there is a relatively flat detachment. In the older cases epi- and subretinal proliferations with corresponding retina deformations can already be found.

The operative procedure takes the above described course: lensectomy is here particularly important, because the lens is frequently adherent to the scar. After lensectomy the ciliary body is examined and completely separated from the scar.

Vitrectomy of the central vitreous and the vitreous in the area of the base will often hardly release the traction on the retina, as the retina is pulled directly by the scar. In any case, before one starts to separate the retina from the scar, the whole vitreous and, if present, central epiretinal membranes have to be removed. Finally, the retina is diathermocoagulated close to the scar and separated from the scar completely bluntly or with the vitrectome (Fig. 18). The hard fibrotic sheet radiating circularly from the scar can mostly, after separation of the retina, be also removed for the greatest part, because it is not connected with the chorioid in the whole length. If this is not possible and if the sheet is very long, it is recommended to cut it through and separate it radially in a few places to avoid future traction through shrinking of the scar.

The tissue that cannot be removed should be carefully coagulated and separated from the retina and the ciliary body. There is, namely, the possibility that newly formed membranes develop through postoperative haemorrhage or fibrin reaction and restore the connection of the scar to the ciliary body and the retina. Redetachment, or even worse, bulbus atrophy through detachment of ciliary body, can be the consequence. The point of this treatment is to reduce the fibrotic tissue of the perforation scar to the smallest possible amount, to separate it from all the surrounding structures and to prevent, by coagulation, possible further activities (haemorrhage, proliferation) (Fig. 19). If this does not succeed, or only partly, and the proliferation becomes active again, at the time of new activity the retina should not be in the immediate vicinity and should be scarred by retinopexy and attached. The ciliary body is,

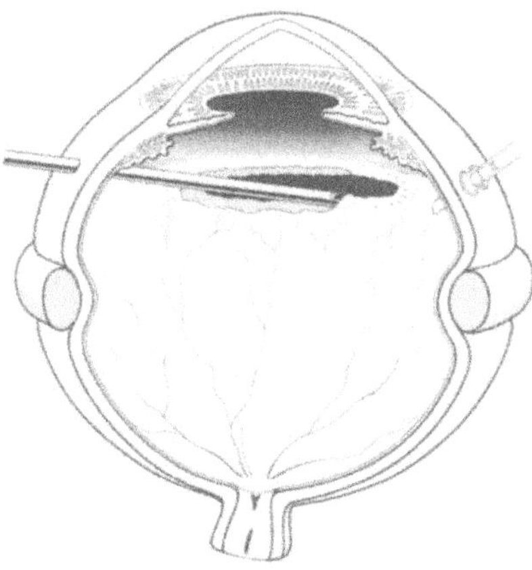

Figure 18. Separating of the retina from the large perforation scar in the periphery.

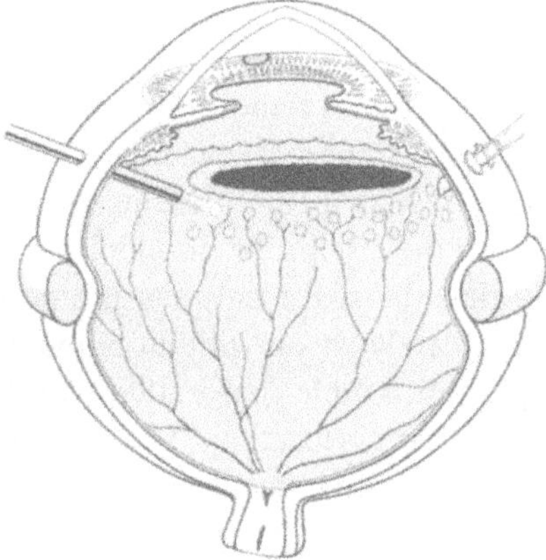

Figure 19. Endolaser photocoagulation after the fixation of the retina with the silicone injection.

as we shall explain later, unfortunately much more difficult to safeguard.

Traction detachment developed after incarceration of the retina occurs mostly after perforation injuries with sharp objects, less frequently after foreign body perforations. It develops after single or double perforations. The epicentre of the detachment is mostly behind the ora, it is characterized by deep incarceration crater and narrow folds. The total traction detachment, frequently combined with the proliferative process, develops in a relatively short time after perforation. The main cause of the detachment – incarceration of the retina – is often combined with the traction on the periphery. The vitreous is mostly detached and fully present, relations in the eye are, through the relatively small perforation wound and small loss of substance, not much disturbed.

(A similar clinical picture, at a smaller scale, sometimes develops after iatrogenic perforation of the retina during the transscleral drainage of the subretinal fluid.)

The operative procedure, after lensectomy and vitrectomy in the above described way, is concentrated on the treatment of the incarceration site and on prevention of reproliferation. The retina completely cleared from the vitreous and the proliferative tissue should be, after diathermocoagulation, separated from the incarceration site. In the beginning we were satisfied with only circumcision of the perforation scar. We found out very soon, though, that after a short time – 1 or 2 weeks – due to fibrin reaction, secondary haemorrhage or reproliferation a new structure develops which connects the perforation scar to the retina again and enables again the traction from the scar on the retina. Since then, we remove about 1 mm of the surrounding retina after circumscribed retinotomy. In this way we create a large distance between the perforation scar and the edge of the retina (Fig. 20).

Retinectomy of the surrounding retina can also be done by diathermo-coagulation. With the diathermy probe the retina is coagulated very strongly in 2–3 rows and the necrotic retina is removed with the back-flush needle. The perforation scar should be cut short and coagulated. After attaching the retina with silicone injection, which as a rule presents no problems, edges of the retina are coagulated with the cryoprobe or endolaser (Fig. 21). It should be mentioned once again that the space between the perforation scar and the retina should be left completely clean, without blood or other debris.

Traction detachment after double perforation with foreign bodies mostly develops some time after the perforation. The period of time between the perforation and appearance of detachment is very much dependent on the size of the foreign body and the destruction developed. With a large and blunt projectile the destruction at the perforation is combined with the contusion effect. The contusion causes a destructive effect on the tissue near the perforation wound and other structures inside the eye. Consequences are haemorrhage, oedema and tearing of various structures (ora, chamber angle). That further impedes healing at the post-traumatic stage and stimulates development of the proliferative process even more. The prognosis in these cases is utterly unfavourable, and every time during primary wound repair and removal of the foreign body it has to be taken into consideration whether silicone oil should be used immediately notwithstanding the existence of retina detachment.

In any case, we are often confronted with cases that recovered after a double perforation with or without removal of the foreign body and only later developed traction detachment. The development of traction detachment, because the rhegmatogenous element is mostly missing, is very slow and develops clearly due to tangential traction from the scar in the posterior pole.

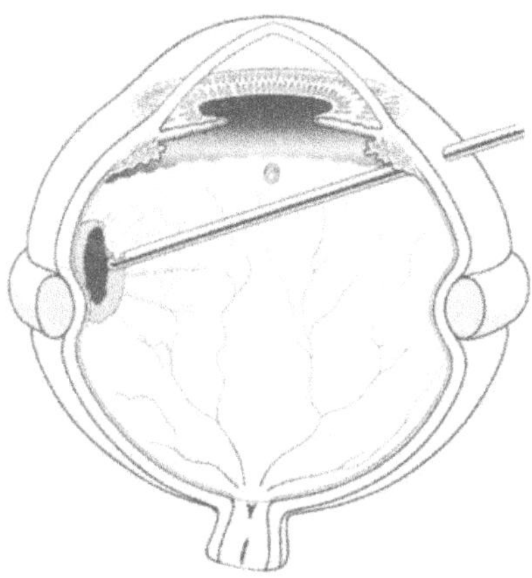

Figure 20. Circumcision of the perforation scar after the retina incarceration.

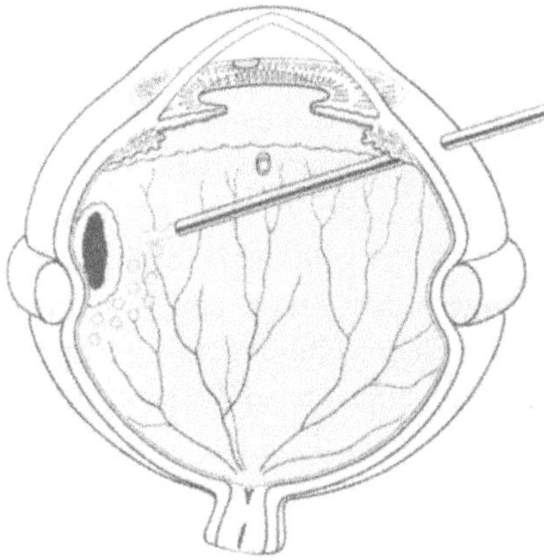

Figure 21. Endolaser photocoagulation of the perforation scar after the fixation of the retina with the silicone injection.

As these eyes are nowadays mostly vitrectomized already during the primary wound repair and have no vitreous, there is no vitreal traction and the entrance site of the perforation does not play such an active role.

Surgical treatment consists usually of lensectomy and vitrectomy, if it has not been done before, with special consideration of the entrance site of the perforation in the anterior segment.

The exit site (causing the traction) is treated as it was described with incarceration, namely with circumcision of the scar and removal of a broad edge of the surrounding retina. As it mostly concerns scars in the posterior pole with thick retinal vessels, the haemostasis with endodiathermy should be performed with greatest care (Fig. 22). (Very unfavourable for such treatment are scars in close vicinity to the disc, which are not so rare. With such scars it is not possible to create enough distance between the scar and the disc, and the process with subsequent traction will very frequently pass around the disc to the opposite retina. Such cases are, unfortunately, mostly given up after repeated operations.)

After circumcision of the scar and careful haemostasis there are no further technical difficulties to be expected. The released and mostly mobile retina can easily be attached with silicone injection. The subretinal fluid is evacuated through the created retinotomy. The attached retina around the perforation scar is coagulated with the endocryoprobe or endolaser (Fig. 23). It should be called to mind once again that the surface between the scar and the retinal edges should be left clean, i.e. without blood and debris at the end of the operation.

Giant tears develop frequently as a late complication of the perforating trauma. With most detachments with a giant tear the latter is found between the equator and the ora, and the mechanism of development is similar to the one with idiopathic giant tears, namely vitreous traction (presumably in a number of cases it has to do with disposition to development of giant tears). Development is frequently, at least in the cases recovered after original trauma, very sudden and dramatic. A small group of giant tears, developed after perforating trauma, are the giant tears in which the retina is torn anterior to the ora. The retinal edge is, contrary to common ora tears, irregular, and an anterior flap is always to be seen. These tears develop slowly through constant traction and develop mostly opposite to the perforation site.

Treatment of these giant tears does not differ from the treatment of idiopathic giant tears and need not be described again. The only addition is that much attention should be paid to the perforation scar. It should be isolated from the retina in the above described way.

Subretinal proliferations developed after perforation are seldom the only cause of traction detachment, not seldom, though, do they dominate the clinical picture. Removal of subretinal proliferation is, therefore, an important surgical procedure, which has to be planned well and performed carefully. For this reason it seems useful to describe this procedure separately.

Basically, subretinal proliferations can only be removed through the retina, so a retinotomy has to be performed. As cutting of the retina is always a serious step, the question has always to be put first whether removal of the subretinal proliferations is really necessary. There are, namely, although in a small percentage, such proliferations which are not relevant for the detachment and it is best to leave them alone.

Subretinal proliferations show, with the exception of circle-formed strands around the disc (napkin ring), no typical clinical pictures so that they could be arranged in groups in one way or another. Seen through the retina, conspic-

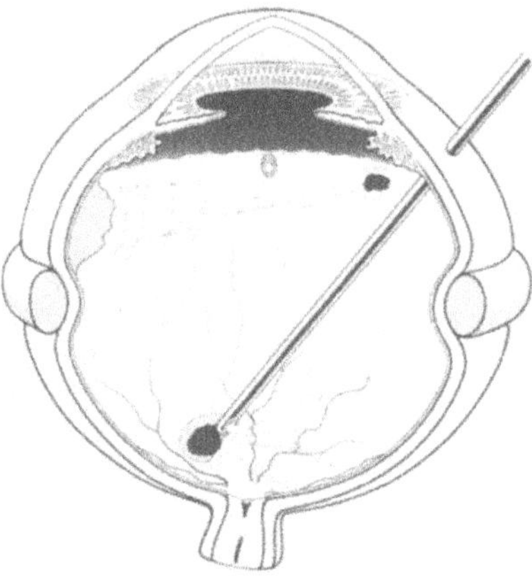

Figure 22. Double perforation – vitreous traction from the entrance site, traction on the retina from the exit site. Circumcision of the scar (performed as the last manipulation after the complete vitrectomy).

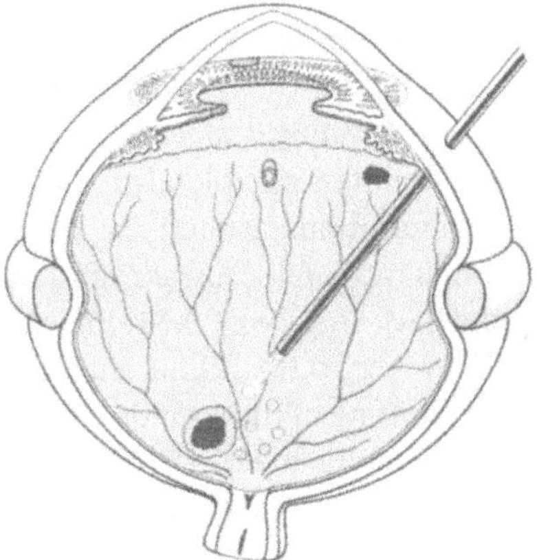

Figure 23. Endolaser photocoagulation of the perforation scar after the fixation of the retina with the silicone injection.

uous are white-yellow strands, which spread in all directions behind the retina and are often in connection with the perforation scar.

These strands spread often in the form of a net under large parts of the retina and are mostly very loosely connected to it. However, these strands are frequently only the most fibrotic parts or edges of sheets, which are less well or entirely not visible through the retina. These sheets are much more adherent to the retina than solitary strands.

All these characteristics are also responsible for various forms of traction and the corresponding look of the detached retina. With solitary strands the retina is smoother and sometimes highly detached in the form of the so-called clothes-line phenomenon. With the subretinal sheets the retina is more folded, and after removal of epiretinal membranes still conspicuously immobile and contracted. Recognizing of various forms of subretinal proliferations is decisive for the choice of surgical technique in which the proliferations are to be removed.

Another fact that could influence the choice is maturity of the membranes. In contrast to the more mature proliferations, which are more white, the fresh proliferations are more brownish yellow and less conspicuous. The sheets are therefore difficult to recognize. Besides, as the membranes are not yet strongly contracted, the retina is much less detached than with the mature membranes. This difference has its clinical meaning, because the new membranes are very fragile and difficult to remove totally.

Removal of subretinal proliferations basically takes place in two ways: through a small, more central retinotomy, or through a large limbus parallel peripheral retinotomy. Both ways have their own indications on basis of the before described clinical features. Solitary strands, clearly visible and presumably removable as a whole are removed through the small central retinotomy. The multiple network strands and sheets had better be removed through the large peripheral retinotomy. Pulling of big proliferations through small central retinotomy has unwanted consequences, because the hole becomes very large and still the proliferations cannot be completely removed. It should be noticed that the circle-formed proliferations around the disc (napkin ring) are not suitable for removal through the small central retinotomy. They are, namely, frequently adherent to the back surface of the retina and therefore break very easily. Because of the adherence to the retina, the release of the traction will not be achieved only by separating of the strands. The very central retinotomy does not offer enough manoeuvre space to peel the strands from the back surface of the retina. If in spite of that one tries to do it, one will notice immediately that the retina tears very easily, because it adheres to the disc.

The place for the central retinotomy is, naturally, decided by the position of the strands. The retina should be cut approximately above the middle of the strands in a place as devoid of vessels as possible. The place is coagulated only once with the diathermy probe, and the middle of the coagulated place is opened with the scissors tip. After that a long blunt spatula is put in the retinotomy and the strand is separated from the back surface of the retina on both sides of the retinotomy as far as possible. After this manoeuvre it can be tried to remove the strand completely. The best instrument is the serated jaws forceps, with which the strand can be grasped well. Pulling should not be done in the direction perpendicular to the retina, because in this way traction on both sides of the strand develops through which it can easily break. It is better to pull the strand with the forceps first on a side parallel to the retinal surface (Fig. 24). Thus traction is exercised on one side of the strand only and the other

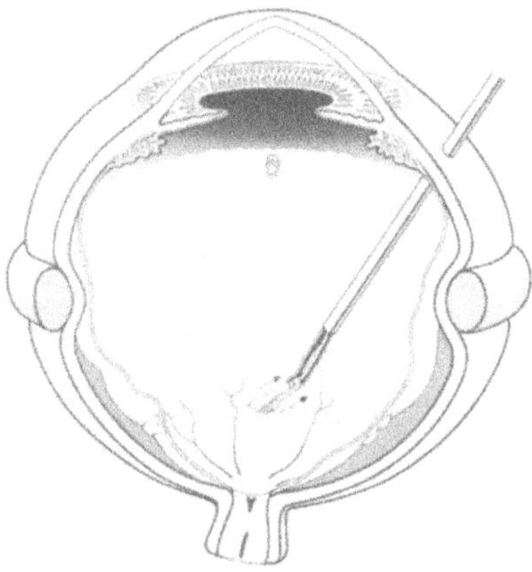

Figure 24. Removal of subretinal strands through the small central retinotomy.

is completely relieved at the same time. The manoeuvre is repeated in the same way pulling at the other side of the strand. In this way there is a greater chance of removing of strand totally, or if it breaks it happens very far from the opening of the retinotomy. Another advantage of this manoeuvre is that the retinotomy opening is not under tension during the pulling and will not be enlarged.

The large peripheral retinotomy offers two great advantages in removal of subretinal proliferations: good view of the back surface of the retina and the possibility of bimanual work in removal of proliferations. With these two advantages the disadvantage of additional work is amply surpassed. The accompanying per- and postoperative complications are not worth mentioning. Indications are all extensive proliferations and certainly immature strands, which are very fragile and cannot be completely removed through the small retinotomy.

The surgical procedure takes place in the following steps. For the purpose of haemostasis and bloodless separation of the retina, a limbus parallel continuous diathermocoagulation of the retinal periphery is performed. One or two rows of coagulates are set as far peripherally as possible parallel to the limbus. One should not hesitate to do it in an area of 180°, because such a large retinotomy guarantees the maximum of comfort and – paradoxically – the minimum of trauma with the intended work. After the coagulation the retina can without difficulty be separated from the periphery, with a blunt instrument or with the sucking power of the vitrectome or the back-flush needle. Once separated from the periphery, the retina is turned over the disc and the retinal back surface examined. Network strand formations are mostly to be removed from the back surface of the retina with a forceps without problems (Fig. 25). With the wide pupil one can work bimanually under the microscope light, so

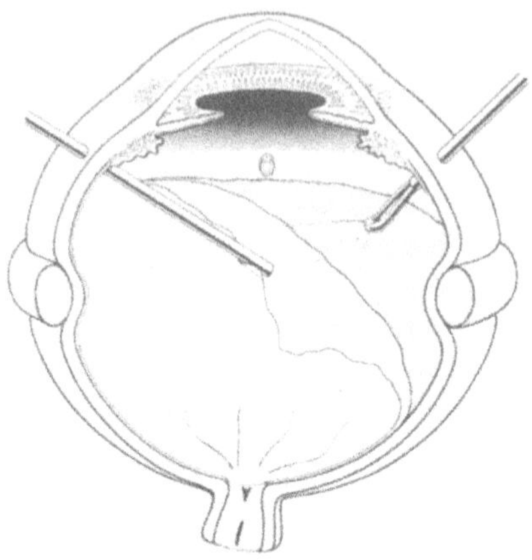

Figure 25. Removal of subretinal proliferations through the large peripheral retinotomy.

that the retina is held in the right position with one instrument, while the strands are removed with the forceps. With sheets, which are sometimes very extensive and cover the whole retina, the bimanual work is a necessity, because the membranes adhere strongly to the retina. In some old cases these membranes can hardly be removed, as they are, particularly centrally, in the vicinity of the disc, very adherent to the retina and besides, hardly distinguishable from the retina in colour and structure.

In such cases great attention should be paid not to perforate the central retina, and therefore it is better to be reserved with removal of these membranes. After removal of the proliferations, when one is already in the retro-retinal space, one should not fail to clean the pigment epithelium from blood and loose pigment. The suitable instrument is the back-flush needle with the silicone brush. After the performed work the always perfectly mobile retina is relatively easy to reattach with silicone injection. In the area of the retinotomy, the retinopexy is performed as usual.

Traction detachment combined with severe damage of the anterior segment is the most serious form of the detachment after the perforating injury. This group of patients has characteristic etiology and course of illness and therefore deserves to be discussed separately. It concerns mostly young people who, almost without exception, have suffered their injuries in a traffic accident. Much too often both eyes are affected and frequently one eye is enucleated immediately after the accident. In these seriously injured eyes the emphasis is always on the damage of the anterior segment, which has been time and again proved disastrous for the further course of the illness. It concerns mostly multiple wounds of the anterior segment with the loss of the greatest part of the contents of the eye (vitreous, lens, iris). These eyes are generally judged in two ways: the most heavily damaged eyes are given up immediately after the primary wound repair or a few weeks afterwards, the less damaged eyes are mostly treated after a few weeks as if the damage has affected only the anterior segment. Mostly irrigation-aspiration procedure is done or cornea graft is performed. Both attitudes are basically wrong, because it concerns the eyes in which the damage in the posterior segment (although not visible) perhaps took place at the time of the accident, and in which a few weeks after the accident that damage is certainly at least as serious as in the anterior segment. A great number of the abandoned eyes from the first group and practically all less damaged eyes from the second group could be saved with a combined radical operation in the anterior and the posterior segment if it were performed shortly after the accident.

In the last 6 years we have operated a fairly great number of such eyes and through this work gained experience and developed a working conception. Describing the operative procedure it should be reported immediately that practically always the only eye patients were concerned. We also think that this procedure, because of great load of work and expenditure of time and very modest results should remain reserved for only this group of patients. As the patients are concerned who have seldom been operated on before, it seems useful to enlighten their case history more closely.

The patients nearly always applied for treatment in either of the two ways characteristic for both groups. The patients with the abandoned eyes were after some time disappointed by unfulfilled promises and conservative treatment and went to look for help by themselves, to a great relief of the helpless attending ophthalmologist. First by change, later more intentionally they came to our clinic. The second group of patients, who were first operated on the anterior segment with reasonable success, was referred to the clinic when complication in the posterior segment appeared, very often after a palliative surgical attempt ('blind' encircling band) in the posterior segment.

For both groups it was common that they applied for treatment after some time, many of them even after a very long time after the accident. The time period varied from 4–5 months to a few years. The eyes were in the pre-phthistic state with expressed hypotony, and the function was reduced to light perception, very often without correct light projection. Ultrasonic measuring of these eyes mostly showed an axis of 14–18 mm, which later proved to relate more to shortening of the destroyed anterior segment and hypotony than to the real atrophy of these eyes. All the eyes examined by ultrasound showed a funnel-shaped detachment. The fundus could not be examined in any of these eyes. Because of a scarred anterior segment the anterior chamber was not existent almost without exception, the iris was mostly not present and the lens was always missing or the lens remnants were incorporated in the scar. The other diagnostic methods, such as electrophysiology, had no worth as preoperative examination, because they were all negative. As it concerned only eyes, the only and absolute contra-indication for the operation was the lack of light perception. After a few operations it proved that the lack of correct light projection was prognostically a bad sign for the functional result at an anatomically successful operation. For a bad anatomic result, or rather for operability of the eye, the time period was of a decisive importance. After $1\frac{1}{2}$ to 2 years after the accident the retina was so changed that unfolding and attachment with the given means were not possible any more. All these facts combined with great expenditure of time needed not only to achieve a positive result but also to abandon such an eye, induced us to reserve this procedure only for the last eyes.

As it is impossible to predict the postoperative results, it is always explained to the patient that a kind of explorative surgery is concerned, in which the possibility and use of further surgery is decided only with the operation, at a certain stage, according to the comprehension and experience of the surgeon. The patient is also told, that even if the functional result surpasses all expectations in the positive sense, the achieved vision in such a damaged eye will probably be of a limited duration.

The operation, which is a cooperation of the anterior and posterior segment surgeons, begins with placing an encircling band and securing of a Flieringa ring. As small corneas are concerned and besides the space must be left free for later sclerotomies a small ring (10–12 mm) is sutured to the exposed sclera. The intention is, after a trephination of the scarred cornea and open sky vitrectomy to insert a Landers keratoprosthesis in the opening of the trephination. For a prosthesis of 6 mm an opening of 5–5.5 mm is trephined, because experience has taught us that the scarred cornea has to be coagulated for haemorrhage and afterwards the opening proves larger than necessary. As there is no normal cornea in these eyes, the trephination is done in the central scar. With the trephine one does not cut through the whole scar, but trephines as deeply as the normal cornea would go and after that the upper part of the scarred cornea is lamellarly separated and removed. Behind this central scar the retina is, namely, always to be found adhering to it, and when the scar is trephined through, it is very probable that at the same time the whole central retina is cut off from the periphery. After having removed the upper part of the central scar, one tries to get to the chamber angle with the spatula at any place at which the cornea does not yet adhere to the scar tissue, and tries to separate the tissue from the corneal backside. At the place where it succeeds, one will frequently notice that the iris is not existent and the tissue to be seen is that of the ciliary body and the ciliary processes. The iris is mostly not to be found, because it was expressed at the perforation.

After removal of the central scar the ciliary body is bluntly dissected from the scar remnants, which is possibe without much trouble and bleeding. (The

92

scar is mostly supplied from the limbus with thick vessels which are coagulated at the edge of the trephination wound, and new vascularization does not pass over to the ciliary body.) After separation of the first part of the ciliary body, the intravitreal space becomes visible, from which some fluid comes. This space is used to circularly separate the scar from the ciliary body, first bluntly with the spatula, then sharply with the sicssors. The retina is sometimes strongly adherent to the scar. At this stage of the operation the retina must be cut under no circumstances, and should be dissected from the scar as intact as possible. The hard fibrotic tissue can, fortunately, be well distinguished from the retina or from the proliferative membranes, and so dissected rather easily. Removal of the central fibrotic scar is a significant moment of the operation, because after that the position of the retina can be judged to some extent. If the retina now falls back and the disc is visible in the open funnel, it is a good sign. A closed funnel with the closely adherent retina is, on the contrary, prognostically bad, although it is not yet the reason to stop the operation.

The following stage is the open sky vitrectomy, in which the peripheral retina should be cleaned and mobilized. The proliferative membranes can, in the beginning, be easily removed with the scissors and a forceps, as long as they are relatively central. Further behind the ciliary body it is always more difficult, especially as the bulbus has collapsed and the ciliary body is lying practically on the retina. To be able to go further is a manoeuvre that is very helpful. First the eye is filled with the infusion fluid and washed for some time. After that the fixation ring is grasped with two forcepses and the ring with the eye is raised as high as possible, so that the whole eye is filled with water. After that, holding the ring with the forcepses, the eye is slowly pushed back, by which the whole water is pressed out. Then the empty eye is again lifted with the forcepses. In this position the retina falls back and separates from the ciliary body, and all membranes and connections between the two become visible and closer at hand. With the assistant's help one can work in this position for a while and clean a part of the periphery. The eye has to be kept wet during the procedure. The open sky vitrectomy should be limited to the removal of proliferations in the area behind the ciliary body and to the mobilization of the peripheral retina. The retina should now be released from membranes and adhesions which connect it to the anterior segment. When this stage has been finished, the Landers keratoprosthesis should be fixed and the further work in the posterior segment done through the pars plana.

If with placing of the Landers keratoprosthesis the trephination opening appears too small, it can be extended with two instruments, e.g. the needle holders, without grasping the edge. The prosthesis is then sutured to the eye with two stitches. The infusion cannula is fastened, if possible, in an area in which there are no scars, and in which it does not easily get stuck behind the retina. If this is not possible the retina is widely cut at this place and, if there is no other possibility, removed. In a great number of cases the 7 mm long cannula is preferable.

By connecting the eye to the infusion and normalizing the pressure the relations in the eye become more normal again. Optically, it is possible to work with the Landers keratoprosthesis. More optically convenient situation can be achieved if a contact lens with methylcellulose is placed above the prosthesis. Judging the situation one tries with vitrectomy to complete that which has not quite succeeded in the open-sky way.

After cleaning of the periphery and mobilizing of the peripheral retina, the central membranes should be removed. As mentioned above, the open funnel and the visible disc is half a guarantee for the success of the operation. Removal of epiretinal and subretinal proliferations, or if necessary, retinal surgery, follows in the above described way. In these cases the necessity of a 360° retinotomy is not rare and the use of retinal tacks with the frequently contracted retina is sometimes also necessary.

The silicone injection follows in the usual way, controlled through the Landers keratoprosthesis. After finishing retinopexy with the cryoprobe or endolaser, the prosthesis is removed, the sclerotomies temporarily closed and the corneal graft sutured. After suturing of the graft the visibility is a little worse than through the prosthesis, but it is still sufficient to refill silicone under visual control and to drain the fluid in front of the disc. As it is understandable, iridectomy at 6 o'clock is not possible in these cases and a contact of silicone with the cornea is difficult to avoid. Yet, if these eyes have not been overfilled with silicone, there is not, at least during the day, a contact between silicone and cornea, because the prominent ciliary body forms with the scar a kind of diaphragm separating the silicone bubble from the cornea.

After having described the successful course, something should be written about the development in the abandoned eyes. They are almost without exception the eyes operated on very long after the accident. In these eyes the first stage of the operation is the same as in the others, and difficulties begin with opening of the funnel. This does not succeed although all epiretinal membranes are removed. If one wants to ascertain, that there are no subretinal proliferations which, perhaps, keep the funnel closed, and performs a peripheral retinotomy, one will find the already described situation. The retina is atrophic, the retinal tissue has partly disappeared and the funnel is actually a thin tube with close running vessels and very little retina among them. In extreme cases this retinal tube is thinner than the diameter of the disc and runs vertically forwards in the same size, passing nearly under the right corner in the peripheral retina, which is still mobile. If such a mushroom is found, with a thin stem longer than 3–4 mm, it means the end of the operation. Every attempt at opening of this funnel is futile in advance, because there is simply no retinal tissue left to centrally cover the bare pigment epithelium.

These eyes have to be abandoned at this stage. The operation is finished with suturing the graft and removing of the encircling band. If possible, instead of a new cornea, the own cornea trephined at the beginning of the operation is sutured, which at least guarantees fast healing of the eye.

With this complicated and time-consuming technique we achieved an anatomic success in approximately 20% of the operated eyes. The functional improvement was also to be noticed with every anatomic success. Unfortunately, in some eyes it was so small, that it had no practical value for the patient. Since the tendency to reproliferation in these eyes is very pronounced, it was very seldom possible to keep the good result, achieved after the first operation. Many eyes had to be operated several times and some of them became blind in the end in spite of the initially good result.

With the detailed description of this unconventional technique and the whole course of illness with these seriously disabled patients it was not our intention only to introduce a new surgical method. We wanted much more to point out that it is possible, although in a small percentage and with modest functional result, even in later stages to achieve something in these severely traumatized eyes. This fact proves that in many of these patients usable vision for the whole life could certainly have been achieved, if they had been operated adequately and in time.

Diabetic traction detachment

The use of silicone oil with diabetic traction detachments depends on severity of proliferative membranes, tendency to bleeding, mobility of the retina and existence of central holes. As most of these factors cannot be judged before the operation, the decision whether or not to use silicone oil is brought during the operation in the majority of cases. For this reason the operative procedure itself at the first stage of the operation is adapted to both possibilities.

The encircling band is placed with diabetic traction detachment for two reasons. In case that silicone oil is used, the encircling band serves to the better presentation of the retinal periphery as with the other indication groups. In case that silicone is not injected, no radical vitrectomy of the vitreous base is performed either. In the postoperative period in these cases a certain contraction of the residual vitreous always occurs, and if there happen to be vitreoretinal adhesions under the opaque vitreous, this contraction of the residual vitreous can lead to retinal tears and subsequent detachment. With an encircling band and circular cryopexy this complication can be avoided.

The problem of lens removal in these patients is a little complicated (not only as far as the decision on the use of silicone is concerned) and has to be discussed more in detail. Led by our experience and by the generally known fact that the pars plana vitrectomy combined with simultaneous lensectomy is, in the diabetics, accompanied with a lot of complications, in the beginning we always tried to preserve the lens in the patients where the silicone had been injected. Yet in a number of patients where the removal of the lens was unavoidable we have noticed that the rubeosis and the haemorrhagic glaucoma did not occur at all. This fact and development of the cataract soon after the operation (particularly in young patients) led us to remove the lens in most patients immediately at the first operation similarly to the other indication groups. The experience of the last 2 years, based on more than a hundred eyes, has shown us that diabetic eyes injected with silicone seldom develop any complications in terms of the rubeosis and haemorrhagic glaucoma. Whether this occurs because the silicone represents a mechanical barrier between the posterior and the anterior segment, or it is due to the stabilizing effect of the silicone by which the unpleasant consequences such as hypotony and inflammatory reaction stay away, remains, for the time being, an open question and need not be discussed here.

So far the group of diabetic traction detachment would not, in our surgical concept, differ from other groups in relation to removal of the lens. Yet there are some considerations that may suggest tackling this problem in a certain number of patients in a different way. The proliferative process in the diabetics has a different biological dynamics and depends largely on the presence of the vitreous. Particularly in elderly patients, recurrence of the proliferation after radical vitrectomy, silicone injection and simultaneous endolaser coagulation is very rare. This fact makes it possible to remove silicone without a great risk in a relatively short time (after 2 or 3 months). Therefore in these patients it is worth considering whether at the operation the lens should not be left in place. If later a cataract should develop in spite of the removal of the silicone, an extracapsular cataract extraction with IOL implantation could be performed.

For all the above discussed reasons, during the operative procedure in diabetic traction detachment the lens should be preserved, in any case at the first stage of the operation. After placing of the encircling band and infusion, one starts vitrectomy with removal of the central vitreous, which is frequently opaque due to haemorrhage. The posterior vitreous is nearly always detached and connected to the retina in various ways. The periphery is mostly free and far removed from the retina and very suitable to vitrectomize without much risk. In this way the posterior vitreous layer is opened first (Fig. 26). Behind the vitreous there is frequently old blood and a drainage of this space makes first the view of the peripheral retina possible and then enables a better orientation and assessment of the whole situation. In easy cases, in which the retina is not detached, the operation ends with removal of the vitreous after separating of vitreoretinal adhesions and possible segmentation of the pro-

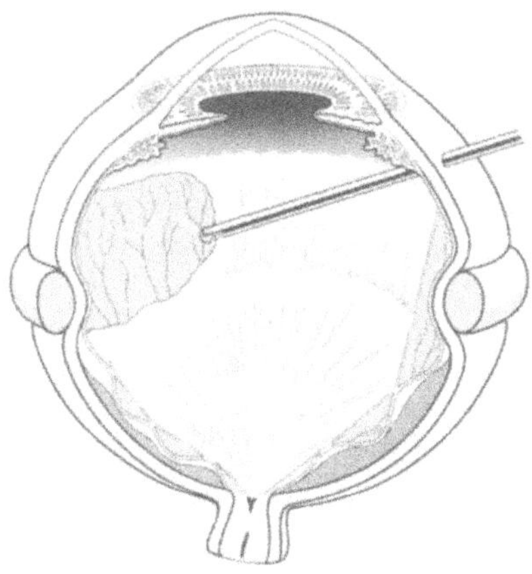

Figure 26. Relieving of the anterior-posterior traction in the diabetic traction detachment.

liferative membranes strongly adherent to the retina. We would prefer, though, to discuss the difficult cases, in which fibrovascular membranes are very massive and in which the retina is totally or subtotally detached and adherent to membranes.

After opening of the posterior vitreous layer and draining of the retro-hyaloid space, the central part of the vitreous, often changed into a vascularized fibrotic membrane, is separated from the periphery. The peripheral vitreous, mostly only haemorrhagic and not much changed, is at this stage removed only so far that it is not optically disturbing. The central vitreous is removed as much as possible and the central edge of the vitreous, which is changed into a fibrotic membrane, is trimmed near to the retina. This fibrotic membrane is mostly – with small breaks – adherent to the retina. The free edge, though, is frequently difficult to separate from the retina, because from this edge a fine transparent membrane very often extends over the retina to the periphery. Before one tries to separate the thick edge of the fibrotic membrane from the retina one should try first to separate this fine membrane from the retina surface. This thin membrane is removed to the edge of the fibrotic membrane and now one can start to separate the fibrotic membrane from the retina. The membrane is very loosely adherent to the retina among the big vessels and can be easily separated with the spatula. Stronger, often point-shaped adhesions, are to be found in the area of the vessels. These adhesions can be separated very well with the motorized scissors. If possible, the fibrotic tissue should not be cut. One tries to separate the whole membrane from the retina more or less bluntly (Fig. 27). In case the pupil is wide, one can also work well with both hands under the microscope light (Fig. 28). Suitable instruments are the endgripping forceps and the blunt or sharp long spatula. With strong adhesions the motorized scissors can be used instead of the

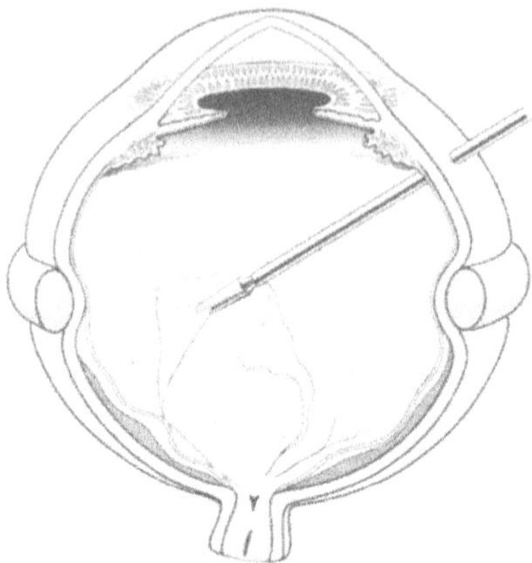

Figure 27. Separating of the fibrovascular membrane from the retina with the forceps.

spatula. With large fan-shaped adhesions and huge membranes it is sometimes also useful to segment the membrane and then to remove it in pieces. In this way the unnecessary perpendicular traction on the retina is avoided, which sometimes occurs with separating of very large membranes which extend outside the vision field of the work. With the removal of small pieces of tissue from the retina, especially if the retina is not or only shallow detached, the horizontal scissors can be used very well. The goal is to remove fibrotic membranes and to completely clean the retina. As situations are very different from case to case, a certain planning in this work is necessary. The released retina is always very mobile and therefore the separating of the last part of membranes is the most difficult. It is particularly difficult in old cases, in which the retina is very atrophic and much thinner than the membrane itself. Tearing of the retina is frequently not quite avoidable and therefore it is best to leave the most difficult parts with the strongest adhesions as the last. With certain experience this is not so difficult to judge. If at the end it is not possible to separate membranes from the retina, it is best to remove the last piece together with the adherent retina (Fig. 29). In this way tearing of the atrophic and mobile retina is avoided and the damage is limited to the retinectomized piece. After the removal of fibrotic membranes from the retina surface, in some cases the fibrotic stalk is left, which is connected to the disc. It should be removed as well. Before removing the stalk one should first make sure that it is not connected to the surrounding retina any more. If the stalk is not free, it should be separated from the retina bluntly with an instrument (e.g. a short spatula). Then it should be grasped with a serrated jaws forceps and separated from the disc with a rotating movement (Fig. 30). Subsequent haemorrhage from the disc, frequent enough, can mostly be stopped with increasing of the intraocular pressure or with injecting some healon.

98

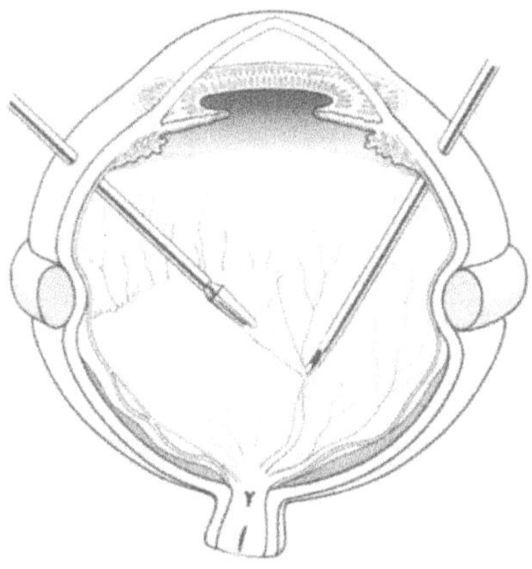

Figure 28. Separating of the fibrotic membranes from the retina with two instruments.

In the described technique of membrane removing heamorrhage is an unpleasant but often unavoidable phenomenon. Haemorrhages from the new vessels of fibrotic membranes are easy to coagulate with diathermy. Haemorrhages from the retina are more disturbing, especially from vitreoretinal adhesions in the area of larger vessels. Although haemorrhages are disturbing during surgery, one should try to coagulate the retina as little as possible before the removing of membranes has been finished. Coagulation makes the retina necrotic and soft so that with traction tears can develop very easily on these sites. Particularly in the beginning of surgery retinal tears are disturbing because membranes have to be handled much more carefully to avoid further tearing of the retina.

During the described surgery the decision ought to be made at a certain moment whether silicone will be injected or not. Reasons for the use of silicone have been mentioned already and should later be discussed in detail. If one has decided to use silicone, one should also decide whether to remove the lens. If it has been decided to remove the lens and to inject silicone, the work with membranes should better be postponed until lensectomy and vitrectomy of the vitreous base has been completed. Vitrectomy of the periphery is simpler if the central retina is still immobilized by membranes. After lensectomy there is mostly also a better visibility, which is very helpful with removing of the membranes. A small disadvantage of this decision is that the pupil sometimes becomes narrow.

Lensectomy is performed in the already described way. Vitrectomy of the vitreous base is relatively simple, because the peripheral retina is attached and the vitreous haemorrhagic. The haemorrhagic vitreous is better visible and can be cut more easily.

In the cases in which one has decided to leave the lens and to inject silicone,

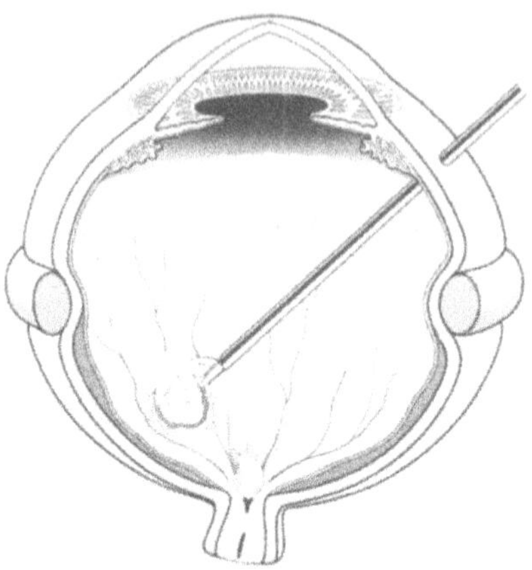

Figure 29. Retinectomy – removal of the retina together with adherent fibrovascular membranes.

vitrectomy of the vitreous base should be undertaken in the same radical way. It is to be accomplished very well with scleral depression and working always on the side of the corresponding sclerotomy, i.e. not across the lens.

After finishing the work in the anterior part of the eye one returns to the posterior part and removes the remaining membranes in the described way. After the removal of fibrotic membranes the retina can be inspected and assessed again. Much more frequently than expected subretinal proliferations are found in difficult diabetic cases. Behind the retina that has been detached for a long time old blood and cholesterol crystals are also frequently found. All that has to be cleared before silicone is injected. After the removal of the membranes there is mostly, somewhere in the central retina, an iatrogenic hole to be found, which can be used for removing of subretinal proliferations. For the same purpose as well as for endodrainage the described retinectomies can be used. After removing of epiretinal and subretinal proliferations, the retina in diabetic eyes is mostly very mobile especially if it was totally detached. In our experience a relaxing retinotomy is never necessary. The so-called shortening of the diabetic retina, which was frequently mentioned and was the reason for bulbus shortening operations in the past, has its cause, in our experience, in the thin epiretinal membranes, already mentioned in the beginning. These membranes probably grow very slowly over the whole retina and are evenly and very closely connected to it without sticking to the retina too strongly. They are very thin, therefore difficult to see and not comparable to PVR membranes, which mostly show an epicentre. Their contraction force is much smaller and equally distributed over the whole retina surface. Because of their transparency they are difficult to observe and as long as they stick to the retina, the retina seems immobile and shortened. It is always recommendable with seemingly immobile retina to look for these membranes, they are

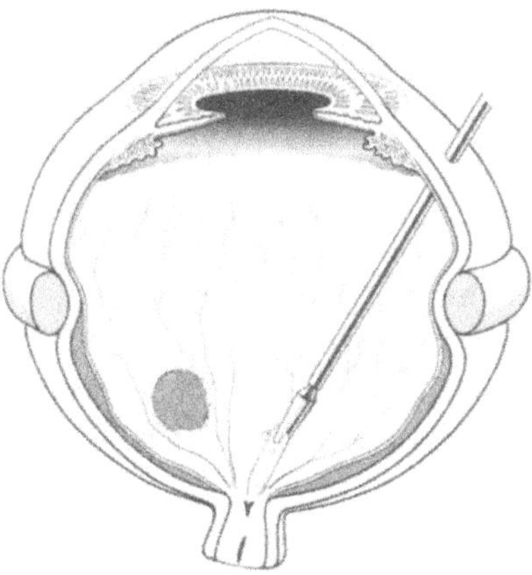

Figure 30. Removal of the central fibrovascular stalk with the forceps.

best recognizable after their shining reflex. After the removal of these membranes the planned retinotomy often proves to be superfluous.

The retina in diabetic patients sometimes shows another kind of contraction. This is the contraction of the retina that has been covered with thick fibrotic membranes for a long time. After the removal of membranes the retina looks like a cast of the removed membranes. Mostly a long-existing process is concerned in which the retina is or has been little or locally detached. Such situations do not develop with total or subtotal detachment, because the traction of the membranes is distributed on the whole retina. With the local traction without detachment in the beginning, the retina is as it were sucked into the membrane by the strong and permanent, slow traction. This bizarre form of the retina under the membrane has to be understood as the result of fight between the traction of the membranes and the adhesion power of the pigment epithelium. (If in this fight tearing of the retina occurs, the rhegmatogenous element is added to the process and the morphology of the retina will change immediately). This retina does not actually need any special treatment and will mostly attach spontaneously in the course of time. Sometimes if there is rather much subretinal liquid under the contracted retina and it cannot be removed in another way, a small retinotomy can be made and the liquid drained. Together with the pressure of silicone during the injection this will help to attach this retina partly. If all membranes are removed, the complete attachment will spontaneously follow in a few days or weeks.

Before one starts to inject silicone, the retina should once again be examined for bleedings. All bleeding sites as well as spontaneously stopped bleeding sites have to be coagulated. As we shall see later, haemorrhages behind the silicone can have very serious consequences and therefore should be prevented.

In most cases treated in this way the retina can be attached by silicone without much trouble. The periphery presents no problems, the central retina is completely mobile and centrally there are always holes that can be used for endodrainage. The exchange liquid – silicone follows quickly and without problems.

At the end of the operation the endolaser light coagulation of the central retina in the form of a panretinal coagulation is always the method of choice (Fig. 31). For the peripheral retina anterior to the buckle one can choose between the endolaser and exocryopexy, depending on the case.

In the end it should be explained when with the diabetic traction detachment silicone should be used and why with the use of silicone the vitrectomy has to be performed so radically.

The use of silicone serves, as mentioned before, to preserve the anatomic situation achieved by vitrectomy. The other aim is to stabilize the eye, by which the unpleasant consequences of the operation, such as hypotony, inflammation, haemorrhage and later rubeosis and haemorrhagic glaucoma are avoided. Therefore the use of silicone with total or subtotal traction detachment with massive fibrovascular membranes and possible central holes is very evident and absolutely indicated. A more local long-existing detachment with a contracted retina after removal of membranes and with central holes also has a much better chance of curing with the silicone injection. A central detachment with a mobile retina can also be cured without silicone, with gas injection and endolaser coagulation, in spite of central holes. The cure rate in these cases without the use of silicone is very high, with silicone it is even higher, and with few cases which recurred after the gas reabsorption, it is regrettable that silicone was not used. There will always remain a large indication group with which both methods can be claimed without feeling of having used the wrong method.

Another controversial indication is the social indication for the use of silicone. In one-eyed patients, namely, in patients who have to leave the hospital directly after the treatment and are difficult to follow-up, in patients with a very bad general condition and in patients with a short life expectation, shortly in general in patients in whom a failure of the operation or a recurrence has serious consequences, the use of silicone is strongly recommended, even in easier cases.

The concept of the surgical technique with the use of silicone differs from the one without in its completeness in removal of the proliferative tissue. We introduced this radical measure into our technique after very negative experiences with the first cases operated with silicone. The patients had been operated on in the usual technique, the membranes had been segmented, the traction relieved and the pieces of the proliferative tissue adhering to the retina left. After a shorter or longer time new proliferations developed from these

102

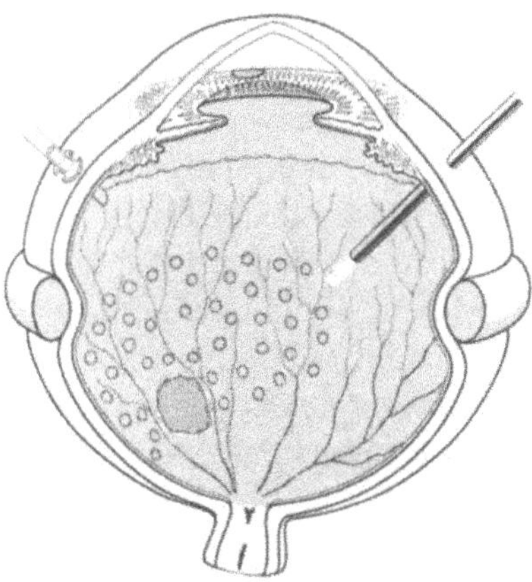

Figure 31. Panretinal photocoagulation of the retina with the endolaser after the fixation of the retina with the silicone injection.

areas. Large holes developed behind the silicone due to newly developed traction and the silicone frequently got behind the retina. The mechanism of this occurrence and our assumptions of the course of the biological process are discussed in detail in the chapter on the postoperative complications. Anyhow, we decided after that to remove the whole proliferative tissue, sometimes at the price of a retinectomy, and in this way to significantly reduce the main basis for new proliferations. The success did not fail to appear and besides, this decision to remove the proliferative tissue at any price enriched our technique in removing of membranes. The fear of making a hole, which with the usual diabetic vitrectomy often paralyses action and sometimes makes it unnecessarily defensive, had disappeared, and with more aggressive surgery we have frequently noticed that some membranes do not adhere to the retina so strongly as it was thought before, and can be removed relatively easily. Removing of all membranes is also faster than segmenting into small tissue islands and can, with certain experience, be even more protecting for the retina. In this way then, all membranes are removed except the tissue stalk on the disc. The following step in the development of the technique was the removal of this mostly vascularized tissue stalk coming from the disc. The basis was the same; with the stalk left we sometimes saw large proliferative sheets which came from it. Naturally, it is not so that therewith the whole problem of reproliferations was solved, but since we started applying this technique the number of reproliferations has been strongly reduced.

Holes in the posterior pole and other indication groups

In this part advantages and disadvantages of vitrectomy combined with the

silicone injection applied in a number of unusual pathoanatomic situations will
be discussed. In this discussion we have confined ourselves to a number of
seldom occuring clinical pictures known to us from experience and do not
intend to claim completeness. It is thoroughly conceivable that there are more
pathoanatomic situations in which silicone can be used.

With the holes in the posterior pole a basic difference should be made
between macular holes without direct traction on the hole itself and those
developed due to direct traction, where the vitreous traction is still present.

Macular holes can certainly be treated without silicone injection and only
with vitrectomy and gas injection (some even without vitrectomy). Use of
silicone comes forward mostly with reoperations when the open hole is combined with the PVR process. The technique does not differ from the one
already described. Removal of the lens is not so weighty in the final result as
with most PVR patients, because in this group mostly highly myopic patients
are concerned. The PVR process is mostly not so extensive and can be treated
in the described way. With the silicone injection the macular hole can be used
for endodrainage. One should take care that the intraocular pressure is not too
high. With too high pressure the drainage of the liquid starts too abruptly, with
a big stream, and the hole is therewith unnecessarily torn and enlarged. The
complete attachment mostly succeeds with the silicone injection without
problems. In highly myopic patients a residual detachment sometimes remains
in the area of the staphyloma and it is very difficult to treat. Mostly additional
small holes are concerned, frequently parapapillar, which, due to absence of
pigment epithelium and non-occurrence of active absorption in the area of the
staphiloma, cannot be attached. As in this area neither the laser nor strong
cryocoagulation can be applied, the only possibility to close these holes would
be the use of the tissue glue.

The traction holes in the posterior pole are mostly seen in highly myopic
patients and are very often combined with total detachment and peripheral
holes. With this complex clinical picture the conventional surgery mostly fails.
Once attempted it frequently only starts the PVR process. Therefore the
combination of vitrectomy and silicone injection is the technique that gives the
greatest chance of success.

The disciform macula degeneration is known as a chronical disease which is
not eligible for surgery. Yet in the past years we have had the opportunity to
treat surgically a few cases of disciform macula degeneration combined with
secondary detachment. Once it concerned the secondary developed subretinal
proliferation with subsequent detachment, four times a massive haemorrhage
was concerned which permeated the vitreous and caused traction detachment
due to shrinkage of the vitreous.

As it is not possible to assess the position of the retina through the cloudy
vitreous, the operation begins with vitrectomy of the central vitreous. The

retina is mostly mobile and centrally adherent to the vitreous. After cleaning of the mobile retina the subretinal haematoma becomes visible. From the first case, with which we evacuated blood and hard bony-like exudate with difficulty and not without damage through the centrally made retinotomy, we have learned that it is much better to make a large temporal peripheral retinotomy and so to inspect and clean the subretinal space without difficulty. After removal of blood and exudates the retina is repositioned and fixed with silicone. The exudate should be removed from the eye before the silicone injection. A few times it was possible to do it with the vitrectome, once it was necessary to remove the solid exudate through the enlarged pars plana incision (Fig. 32). The functional result with all cases was limited to improvement of the peripheral visual field. A big central absolute scotoma, which could be observed with the cases postoperatively, suggests that the retina was so damaged even before the detachment and that an operation with the cases without detachment would not bring functional improvement.

The next group are the pathoanatomical changes developed as early or late consequences of an acute disease of the eye. The retina is locally affected during the course of the disease, and the proliferative process develops later, sometimes in an atypical form. The use of silicone serves more to preservation of the anatomical situation and to prevention of the proliferative process.

The eyes with the bacterial endophthalmitis which are not vitrectomized in time sometimes, during surgery, show retinal detachment and great, often central, holes due to the retinal necrosis. Silicone injection after the complete vitrectomy and lensectomy can rescue some of these severely damaged eyes.

With the mycotic endophthalmitis, which has a more chronic course and is often treated conservatively, the organizing of the preretinal exudates and a slowly developed traction detachment occur at a later cicatricial stage. At this stage the vitreous is not so infiltrated any more and actually does not necessitate vitrectomy, which is more required by the increasing traction detachment. After vitrectomy, which gives no problems, one is confronted with completely different membranes from those with the PVR or diabetic retinopathy. They are hard, for the greatest part strongly adherent to the retina and frequently not to be separated from it. With much caution one sometimes cuts out lamellarly from the retina using two instruments. That is frequently necessary too, because the adhesions are frequently close to the macula or the disc, which does not allow removing of the retina together with the membranes. On the nasal side a retinectomy is then easier to perform and if necessary the retina with the membrane can be removed at the same time. Injecting of silicone and attachment of the retina follow in the usual way.

The acute retina necrosis is also a clinical picture with which, at a later stage, large tears and secondary detachment occur. The vitreous is frequently much infiltrated and the situation of the retina can be judged well only after vitrec-

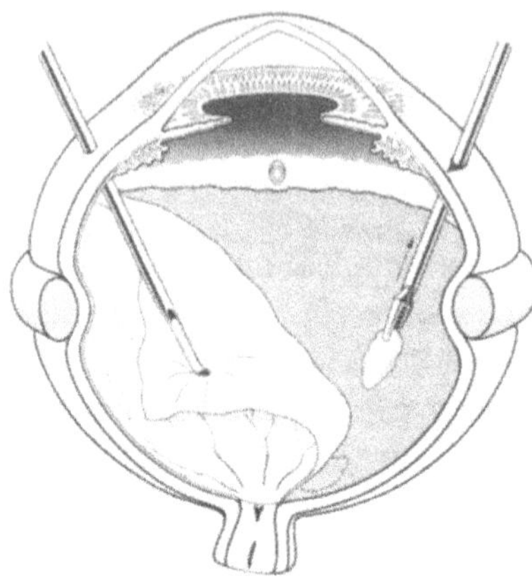

Figure 32. Removal of the solid exudate in the DMD with the forceps after the large peripheral retinotomy.

tomy. The tears develop because of disappearance of the peripheral retina. The retinal parenchyma has peripherally totally disappeared and the peripheral part consists only of the net of closed vessels, through which the subretinal liquid can be drained. At the beginning of the detachment the central retina is mostly completely mobile and looks relatively normal. Due to the peripheral necrosis giant tears of 360° can someties develop. After vitrectomy and removal of the peripheral retina remnants the retina is attached without problem by silicone.

While the use of silicone in the described pathoanatomic situations developed after an acute illness leads to relatively good anatomical and functional results, the results in the situations developed after chronic diseases are less gratifying. We mean here secondary traction detachments with the morbus Eales, morbus Coats, and various forms of uveitis of unknown etiology. Although with these diseases a simple vitrectomy possibly combined with photocoagulation has a good result at an early stage, when there is no detachment yet, and seldom leads to complications; at a later stage, when the proliferative process has already caused traction detachment, the success of vitrectomy is very dubious, sometimes even stimulating for the whole process. The silicone injection changes hardly anything in this situation. These eyes are mostly very hypotonic, the process is progressing under the silicone and reoperations are frequently necessary. During surgery removal of the membranes is very difficult, they are multi-layered, difficult to recognize and little structured. In the older cases, on the contrary, the membranes and scars in the area of the ciliary body are sometimes strongly organized and difficult or not to be removed at all.

The main difficulty in treatment of these eyes is that the biological problem leading to this exudative proliferative process is anatomically even more difficult to localize than with the PVR process or diabetic retinopathy. This fact makes application of surgery as therapy with these cases even more questionable, less promising, than with other indications. It certainly holds even more for the retinal surgery as its most radical form. These are frequently very unpleasant operations, with which at the end one does not know exactly what has been achieved with the operation, and the postoperative course is not much better either. All this forces us to the conclusion that in these cases one has to be rather reserved with radical surgery and the use of silicone, the more so because in these cases surprisingly good results can often be achieved with conventional buckle techniques and cryocoagulation and these should be tried first.

A few words have to be said yet on the sad problem of ROP children. It is not our intention to discuss in detail the surgery of the cicatricial stage of ROP, we only want to discuss in short the use of silicone combined with the retinal surgery.

With the severe form of the ROP detachment, at the fifth cicatricial stage, the greatest problem after opening of the funnel and removing of a part or the whole of the fibrotic scar is mobilizing of the retina. The retina is stiff, completely contracted and pulled forward into a sagital fold (anterior loop traction). The use of silicone as an instrument mostly also fails due to this stiffness of the retina, because the silicone gets behind the retina through the retinal holes or if they are not there through the most detached pars plana. If this does not happen and the subretinal liquid partially drains itself behind the pars plana, the sagital fold is pressed to the bulbus wall and so a radial shortening of the retina with residual central detachment develops. To prevent this, in some cases we retinotomized the retina centrally from the sagital fold and attached the retina without much trouble. However, this later resulted in a complete disaster, because shortly after the operation the retina contracted and shrunk until it was not more than a lump in front of the disc. The reoperations undertaken before this final stage ended in the same result. From our own experience and occasionally examining the children who had been operated on in the same way somewhere else, we decided not to use silicone and particularly not to perform retinal surgery as the first operation in these cases. The retina of the premature babies is probably so changed or un-developed that it reacts in a different way from the full-grown retina, which makes it completely unsuitable for this kind of surgery. The use of silicone can be useful with the second operation, when due to spontaneous mobilization of the retina the retinal surgery is not necessary, or with the secondary detach-ments, which represents a completely different situation.

Plate 5. Traction detachment after perforating trauma.

1. Dubble perforation with I.O.F.B. Traction detachment due to traction from the exit site 1 year after the perforation.
2. Vitrectomy, circumcision of the perforating scar. Silicone tamponade.
3. Subretinal proliferation in the nasal part after the dubble perforation. In the foreground traction on the vitreous base.
4. The same case. The exit of subretinal proliferation in the perforation scar.
5. Situation after the operation (vitrectomy, lensectomy, large peripheral retinotomy, removal of subretinal proliferations, silicone tamponade) and after the removal of silicone.
6. Idem.

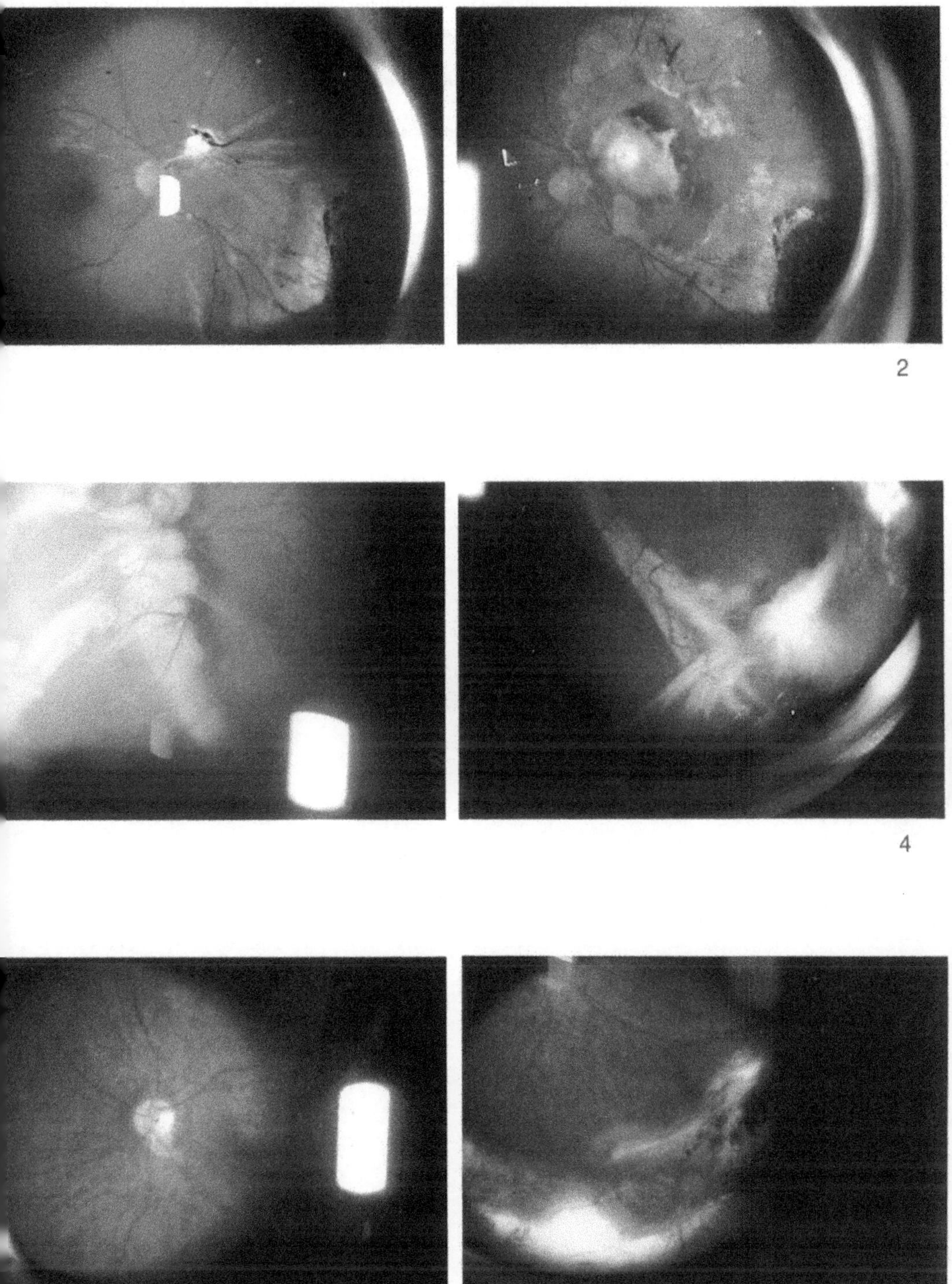
2
4
6

Plate 6. Perforating trauma – traction detachment combined with severe damage of the anterior segment.

1. Prephthisis – an only eye 15 months after the trauma.
2. Removal of the scar.
3. Situation after open sky vitrectomy. The retina is visible in the trepanation opening and was adherent to the scar.
4. Placing of the Landers keratoprosthesis.
5. Postoperative situation of the anterior segment.
6. Postoperative view of the fundus. Satisfying anatomic success. Very small improvement of function.

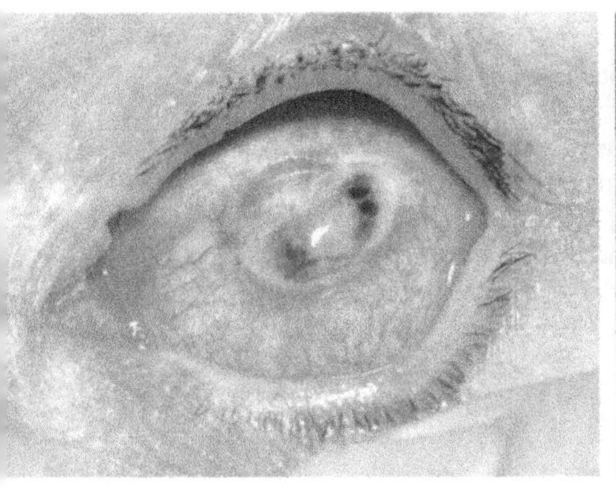
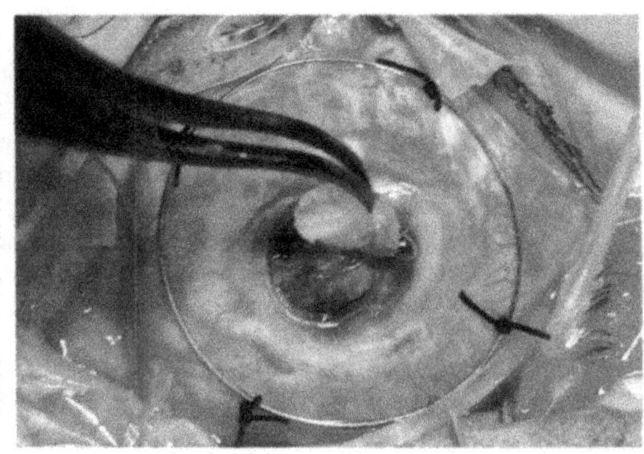

2

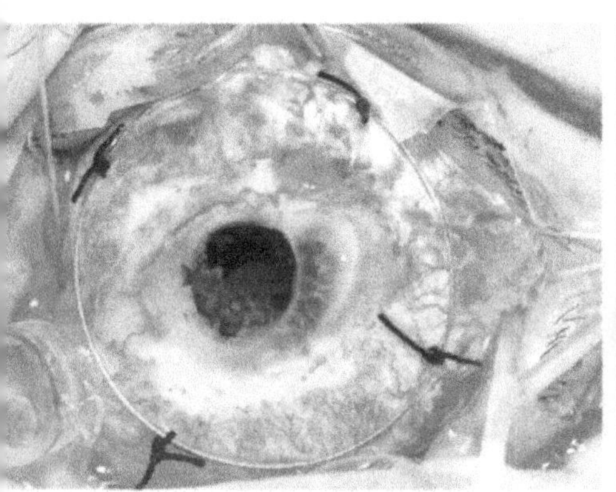
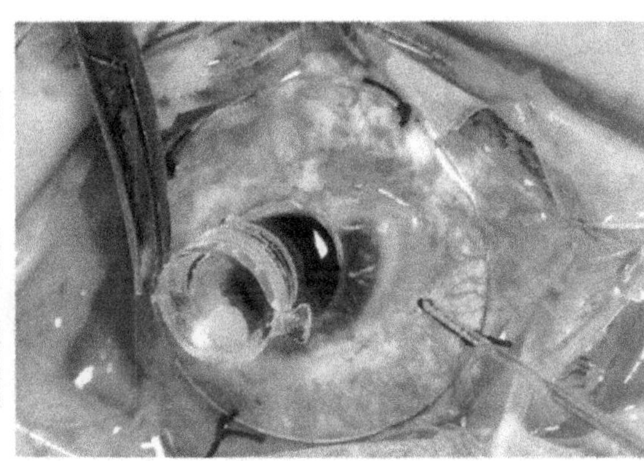

4

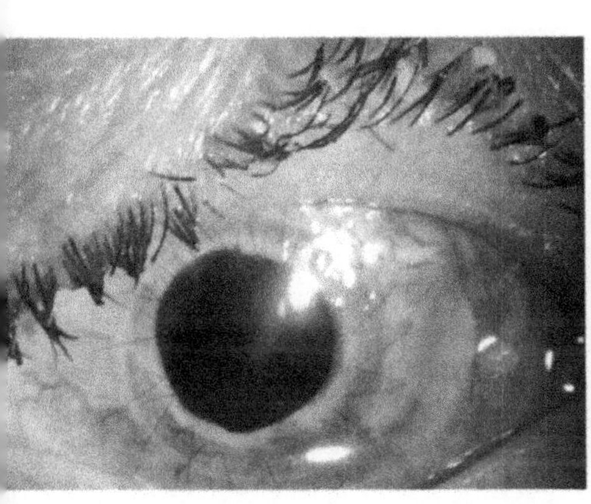
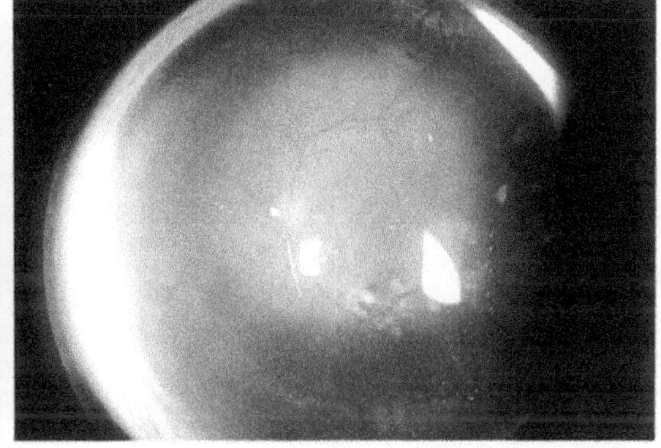

6

Plate 7. Secondary traction detachment of various etiologies.

1. Massive fibrovascular membranes and a total traction detachment in proliferative diabetic retinopathy.
2. Situation after vitrectomy, complete removal of membranes and silicone tamponade.
3. Proliferative traction detachment after Candida endophthalmitis.
4. Situation after the operation: vitrectomy, silicone tamponade, retinectomy. Nasally an iatrogenic hole after removal of adherent membranes with the retina. Endocryopexy.
5. Situation after the operation of the secondary fraction detachment in a case of disciform macula degeneration with massive subretinal haemorrhage. Vitrectomy, retinotomy, silicone tamponade.
6. The same case. A bone-like substrate of D.M.D. removed through the retinotomy and enlarged sclerotomy.

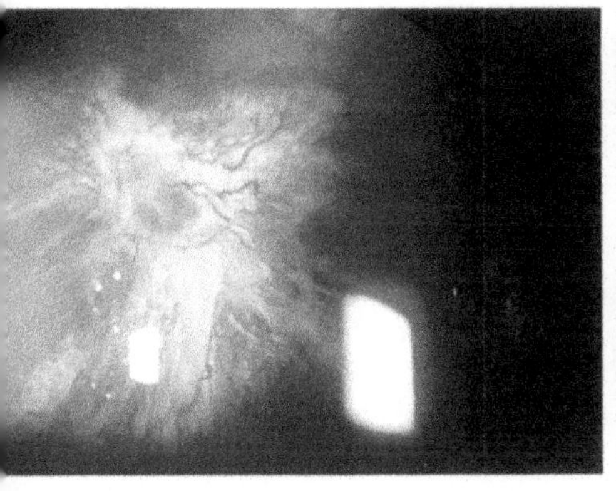
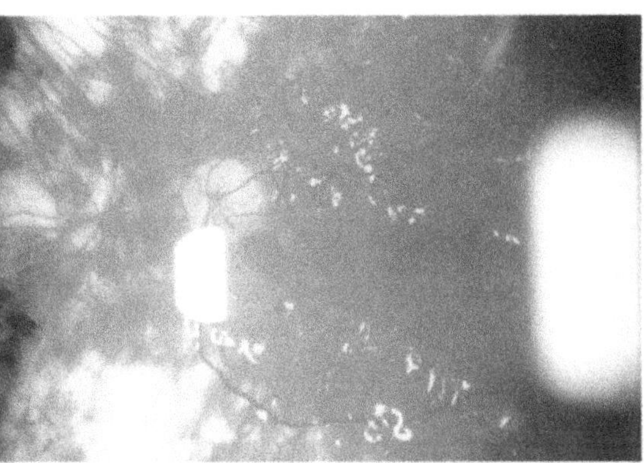

2

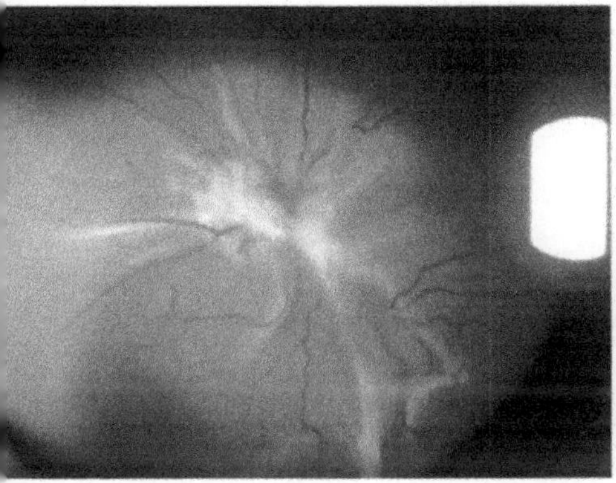
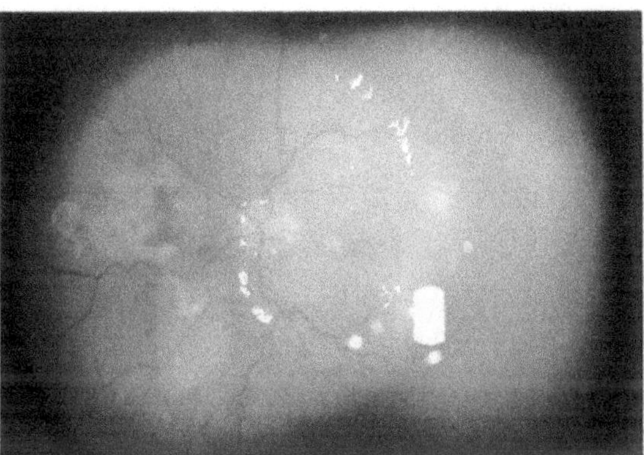

4

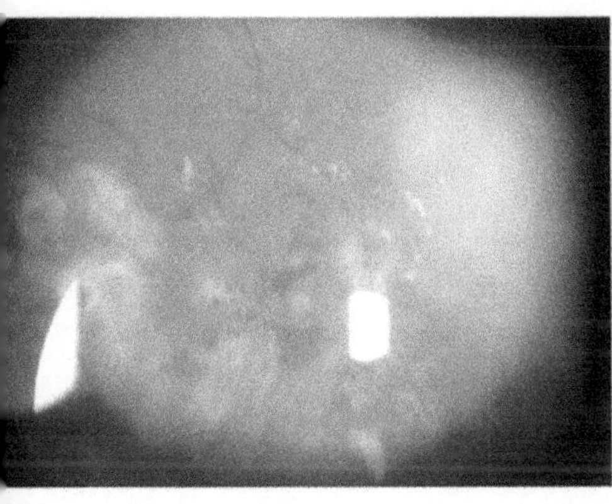
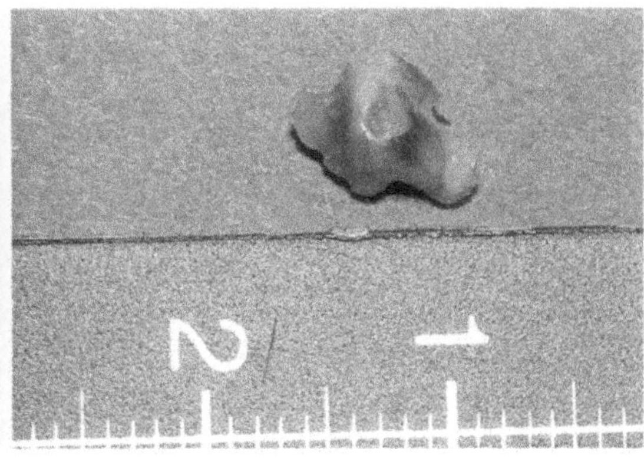

6

6. Peroperative complications

Peroperative complications with this complex and aggressive technique are very frequent and ought to be discussed in detail. They mostly develop because of inexperience of the surgeon and the wrong planning of various manipulations in the operative procedure. When we started with this surgery, without experience and without the surgical concept, looking for surgical solutions in difficult cases, we often had to spend up to 50% of the operating time on treatment and surpassing of peroperative complictions that, for the greatest part, we had caused ourselves. Non-appearance of many complications is not only due to surgical experience and controlling of the instruments but much more to the insight in the given situation and the consequent operative planning. A certain number of peroperative complications, though, is not to be avoided. We are going to discuss them so as they occur in the normal course of the operation.

The complications with insertion of infusion are in so far specific for this technique as they concern many cases which are extremely hypotonic, and in which the pars plana is also detached. The possibility for the infusion cannula to get under the retina or the chorioid is very real and the cannula must be well under control. In dubious cases it is recommendable, as already mentioned, to take the extra long, 7 mm cannula.

In lensectomy it may sometimes occur that the hard nucleus falls backwards through the open lens capsula. If the retina is immobile and covered with membranes, it is mostly possible to remove the nucleus with the vitrectome without damaging the retina. If the nucleus is too hard, it can be pulverized with the endodiathermy probe and then removed with the vitrectome (Fig. 1). Another possibility is to crush the nucleus with the forceps and suck off the small pieces with the back-flush needle or the vitrectome (Fig. 2). Both manipulations take rather much time and patience, but they are relatively safe for the immobile retina. The situation is different if the retina is mobile and the detachment more bullous. As it is very easily possible to seriously damage the retina with the vitrectome and other instruments during the manipulation, it is

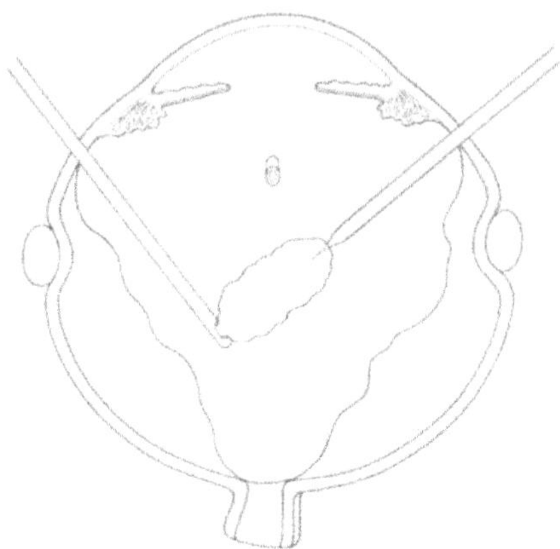

Figure 1. Crushing and removing of the lens nucleus with the diathermy probe and the vitrectome.

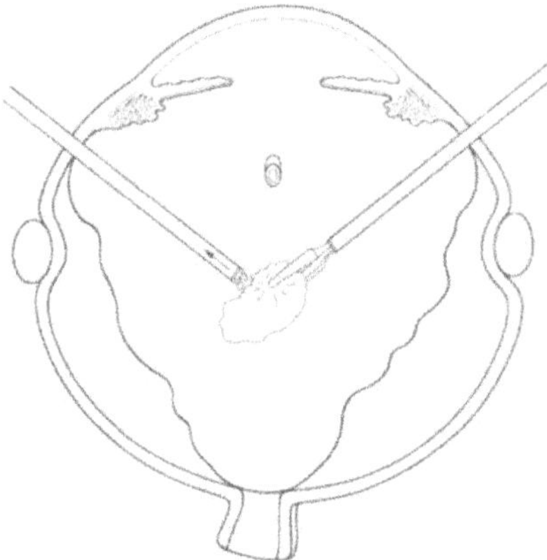

Figure 2. Crushing and removing of the lens nucleus with the back-flush needle.

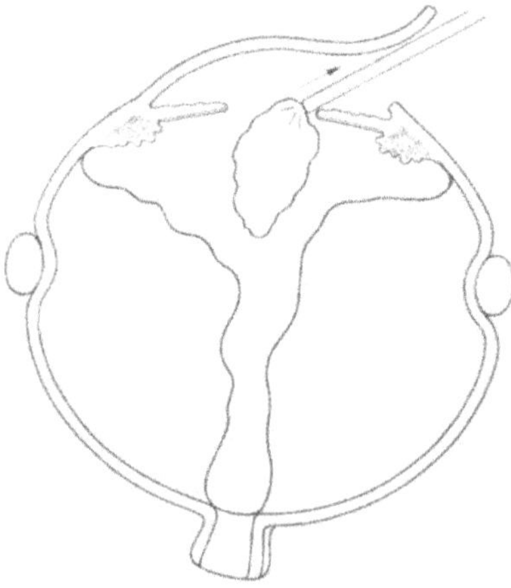

Figure 3. Removing of the lens nucleus ab externo through the corneal wound.

better to extract the nucleus through the cornea ab externo with the cryoprobe (Fig. 3).

After vitrectomy of the periphery and the area of the vitreous base, it may happen (particularly if the pars plana is detached) that first the residual vitreous fibrillae and subsequently the peripheral retina becomes incarcerated in the sclerotomy. It is almost unavoidable in some eyes with the frequent exchange of the instruments and sometimes a too high intraocular pressure (Figs. 4 and 5). In case of an incarceration first intraocular pressure should be decreased and then through the other sclerotomy one should try to pull the retina out of the sclerotomy sucking it with the vitrectome. Afterwards one should try to remove the vitreous completely from this area so as to prevent a new incarceration. This will not succeed completely in most cases, and after a while the retina will come again in the sclerotomy. The final solution is the retinectomy with the vitrectome from the other sclerotomy, in the course of which the retina together with the vitreous is removed from this area. Figs. 6 and 7). The size and right place of the retinectomy is controlled with the scleral depression of the sclerotomy area.

Bleedings from the sclerotomy sometimes occur in reoperations and can be very unpleasant. They are not to be underestimated and should best be treated immediately. If it does not succeed to present the sclerotomy site from outside with scleral depression and coagulate it, it is best to close it with a suture and to make a new one.

During the vitrectomy of the zonula fibres or the vitreous base it can happen that the ciliary body or the chorioid are damaged with the vitrectome. These bleedings are not very strong and can be localized well with scleral depression and then coagulated. If, exceptionally, they are very strong (chorioid) then, besides indentation the combined back-flush needle with diathermy is very helpful, because at the same time one can suck off the blood and coagulate the place after having localized it. Bleedings from the peripheral retina occur either through the vitrectome, or through removal of peripheral membranes and tearing of the retina. Stopping the bleeding is mostly without problems, because the vessels are small and the bleeding spots clearly visible.

This is not the case if it concerns retinal haemorrhages from the post-equatorial retina, where the vessels are much stronger and may bleed heavily. The iatrogenic bleedings and tears are though rare in this area and the places of the planned retinotomies should always be coagulated in advance. With the diabetics the central haemorrhages at removal of epiretinal fibrovascular membranes are very frequent and unavoidable. However, as it has been described, one should be very cautious with coagulation as long as one still has to pull at the retina, and indeed coagulate only the indispensable places. Retinal bleedings from the edges of retinotomies or tears are very frequent after cryocoagulation due to subsequent hyperaemia of the retinal vessels.

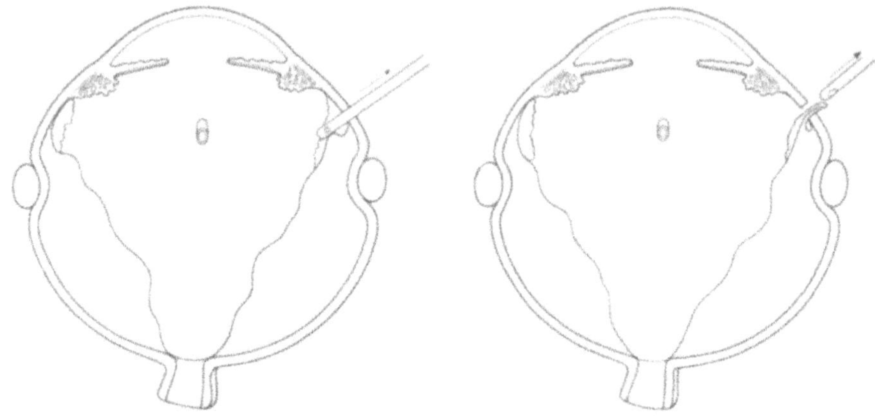

Figs. 4 and 5. The vitreous and the retina incarceration in the sclerotomy with the exchange of the instruments.

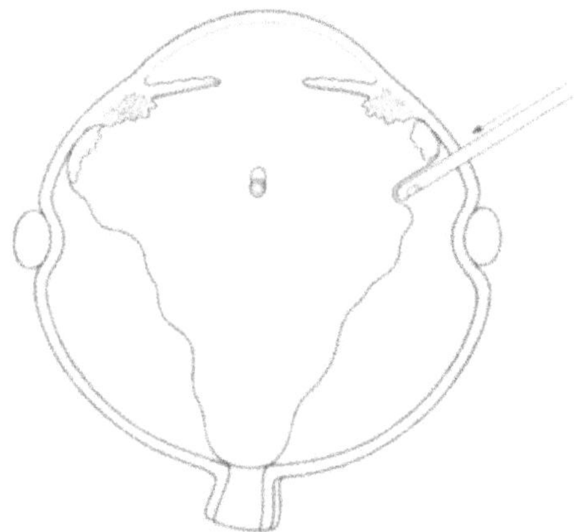

Figure 6. Getting of the vitrectome behind the retina.

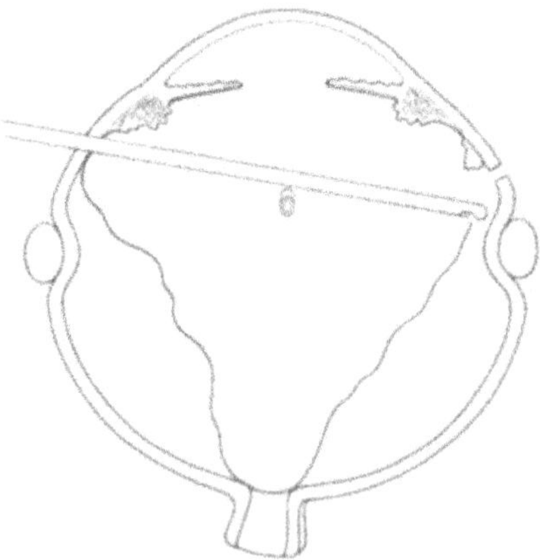

Figure 7. Retinectomy – removal of the retina in the vicinity of the sclerotomy.

They should be coagulated immediately to prevent blood coming under the retina in greater amount. As first aid with such bleedings, before one can coagulate, the intraocular pressure should be increased immediately. These unpleasant complications of cryopexy are largely avoided by using endolaser coagulation.

Bleedings from the chorioid are not frequent centrally but the more unpleasant and sometimes serious. Iatrogenic bleedings develop during endodrainage through the central retinotomy, if one manipulates with the back-flush needle uncautiously and damages the chorioid. This is nearly completely avoidable if the cannula with the silicone tip is used for this purpose. Further, chorioidal bleedings are seen at manipulations with the instruments near or on the chorioretinal scars. These bleedings are mostly easy to localize, especially if the retina has been cut before (which is often the case) and they are easy to coagulate.

The chorioidal haemorrhages from the posterior pole in the highly myopic eyes operated several times are very rare, we have seen them twice. These haemorrages develop almost spontaneously, i.e. also in very careful dealing with instruments; they are very heavy and sometimes difficult to localize. Nevertheless in one such case it was not possible to stop the haemorrhage and the eye had to be abandoned. It concerns a kind of abortive explosive bleeding, which is better visible through the performed retinotomy and possible to localize to a certain extent.

Typical explosive chorioidal haemorrhage developing spontaneously at another stage of the operation is very rare. It is not caused directly by manipulation with the instruments, develops apparently without cause, is only indirectly noticeable and therefore difficult to localize. In this situation it is best to increase the intraocular pressure, to close the sclerotomies and to stop the operation. The eye should then be operated again soon afterwards, in 2 or 3 days. The cause of the haemorrhage can be mostly explained after the operation through the analysis of the course of the operation and the anaesthesia and the internal condition of the patient. Haemorrhages from the disc are very rare, with the exception of the diabetic patients. In the diabetic eyes haemorrhages develop, as it has been described, after the removal of the proliferative stalk from the disc. These bleedings require no treatment and mostly stop spontaneously.

A few things about the retinal tears have been said when dealing with the operative techniques and there is not much more to be said either. Basically, this complication can be overcome and it is certainly not one that has to be specially treated. Yet, it is certainly so that one has to avoid making tears, and if they have to be made, then it is much better not to do so at the beginning of the operation. Every small retinal tear can become larger with long and uncautious manipulating. A large tear, especially central, means not only loss of the valuable retinal parenchym, but presents also an additional difficulty with attachment of the retina at the end of the operation.

Radial and circular buckles in all preoperated eyes can sometimes be an obstruction for the course of the operation. Removal of the membranes in the corners between the buckles can be difficult, and a too strong circular buckle can optically obstruct the view of the central retina immediately behind it. Finally, too strong indentation can make unfolding and attachment of the retina with the silicone injection more difficult. Therefore it is sometimes necessary to remove the buckles or to cut the encircling band. On the other hand, the pre-existing tears are indented and closed with the buckles and it is a great advantage to keep these tears closed at the first stage of the operation. Therefore it is best to find the radial buckles before vitrectomy and to open the Tenon capsula above the buckle and prepare it for extraction. In this way such a buckle can always be removed without problems with the forceps when necessary. Sometimes it has to be done during removal of the central membranes, much more frequently during the silicone injection. The encircling band can be divided also before vitrectomy, it need not be removed. In some cases, though, the encircling band has intruded the bulbus wall so that it is difficult, time-consuming and also risky to expose it. In such a situation, when the encircling band has cut through the whole chorioid, it is possible to cut it from inside. It is only necessary to coagulate the retina on the buckle of the encircling band and to divide the encircling band with the scissors or the Sato knife (Fig. 8). Elastic, hard silicone will retract and the indentation will immediately diminish under the intraocular pressure.

A frequent peroperative complication, which although avoidable happens again and again, is migration of silicone oil under the retina. Basically it can occur only when the retina is under tension. Nearly always it is combined with a pre-existing hole in the retina, very seldom in this technique is that the intact retina is torn during the silicone injection. Tearing of the retina by expansion power of the silicone happens much easier and much more frequently with the use of silicone oil as instrument for separating membranes from the retina. If this occurs through a central hole it is immediately noticed,because the hole suddenly becomes larger, with tense edges, and if the retina is not much lifted, the glossy reflex from the contact with the chorioid is observed. If the hole is in the periphery and outside the visual field, the occurrence is not noticed immediately. Only a little later it is noticeable on the behaviour of the retina. First no flattening of the retina is seen any more and immediately afterwards an increasing detachment is seen in a part of the fundus. With the thin retina the silicone bubble is also recognizable. The first that has to be done is to stop injecting of the silicone and to examine the situation. Evacuation of the silicone from under the retina should not be started before the cause of this complication has been discovered. With a detailed examination it is always

120

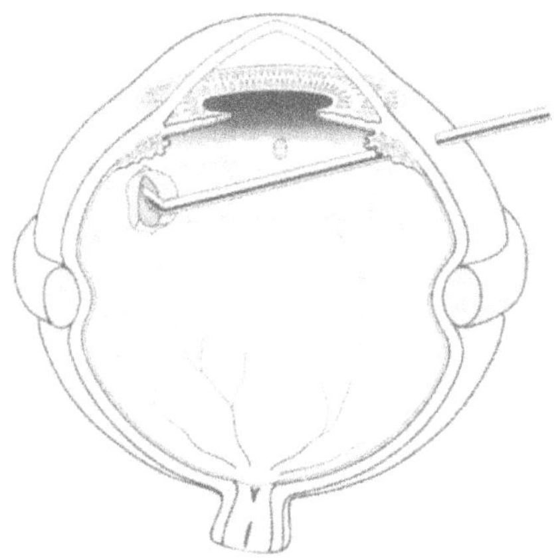

Figure 8. Dividing of the encircling band from inside.

found, and originates as always in the immobility of the retina. It is again, as always, the consequence of insufficiently released traction. Epiretinal or subretinal proliferations, less frequently vitreoretinal contraction are mostly the causes. As far as remaining epiretinal membranes are concerned it is even easier to remove them from a retina stretched by the underlying silicone. Only then the silicone should be removed. If a retinotomy is chosen as solution, it is also better to perform it before evacuating the silicone. If a larger retinotomy is needed, the complication will be solved by itself, because the underlying silicone will join the large bubble in the intravitreal space through the retinotomy opening. It should be noticed that with every manipulation the intraocular pressure ought to be very low, otherwise with every pull on the retina even more silicone will come under it.

In the described situation, the silicone comes under the retina during the injection and the retina plays a passive role. If not noticed in time, a great amount of silicone can thereby get under the retina.

Another possibility to get silicone under the retina is when operating under the silicone and manipulating with the retina. In this situation there is a constant intraocular pressure. The silicone is not injected at the moment, but the retina is pulled at (e.g. removal of membranes, cutting of the retina). With a movement exaggerated for the given situation the retina is lifted too fast or too far and at this moment the silicone comes under the retina. The amount of the silicone is therewith mostly relatively small. The same can also happen with diathermo- or cryocoagulation, if the probe is lifted too fast when the retina still sticks to it.

After one has assured that the retina is not under traction any more, one should try to evacuate the silicone. This can be done in three different ways. The choice of the technique for evacuation of the silicone depends on the amount of silicone under the retina.

121

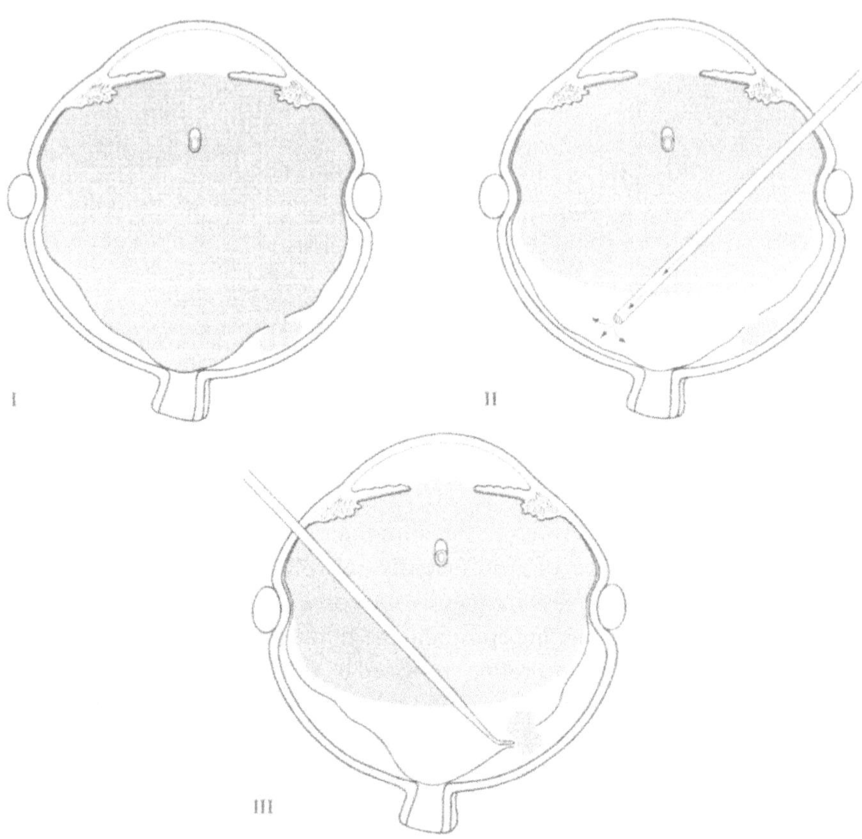

Figure 9. Removal of the small silicone bubble behind the retina; I, II, III: After the injection of the Ringer solution, by which the main silicone bubble is separated from the small one, the small silicone bubble is squeezed out with the spatula through the hole in the vitreal space.

With small amounts (mostly a small bubble which has come backwards through a central hole) it is best to inject some Ringer solution in front of the disc, after letting out a little silicone to decrease the intraocular pressure. The large silicone bubble is moved upwards in this way and loses contact with the small bubble behind the retina. After that the small bubble, tending to float upwards anyhow, is easily pressed with the spatula through the hole into the intravitreal space (Fig. 9 I, II, III).

The second technique is to be applied if larger amounts of silicone are concerned and the silicone bubble is much larger than the hole. Again, the intraocular pressure has to be decreased and after that one ought to enter the hole with the cannula that has a side opening and is attached to the silicone suction pump (or the sucking device or the vitrectome) and slowly suck out the silicone bubble (Fig. 10 I, II).

122

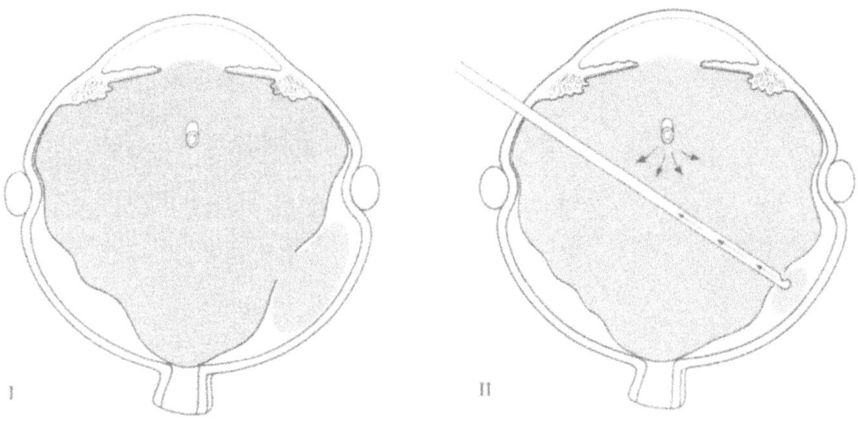

Figure 10. I, II. Removal of the bigger silicone bubble behind the retina.
The bubble is sucked out with the cannula with a side opening.
Simultaneously silicone is injected and the retina attached.

Good visibility is very important therewith, because during the sucking out the cannula opening should stay in contact with the silicone. The sucking power of the device is adapted to the sucking of viscous silicone and if the contact with the silicone is lost, the device can damage the retina.

The third technique is suitable to be used in the situation with very much silicone under the retina, which has mostly come behind through a peripheral hole. The best to be done in such a situation is to perform a long peripheral retinotomy through which the silicone from the back can escape into the intravitreal space. Simultaneously the whole silicone should be removed from the eye. Attachment of the cut retina is much easier if silicone is injected again in the familiar way (Fig. 11 I, II, III).

In the end the complications should be described which make the visibility and normal surgery more difficult.

Haziness of the epithelium is a complication which, with the use of mobile contact lens with methylcellulose, does not frequently occur. The usual abrasion of the epithelium is, in this case, the best solution.

A purely optical disturbance occurs very frequently when operating with silicone in aphakic eyes. After some time, due to changing of the intraocular pressure, the anterior chamber becomes a little shallower and the silicone prolapses to the anterior chamber through the pupillary opening. Therewith, particularly if the pupil is half-wide, a disturbing astigmatism of the silicone bubble develops and the fundus picture becomes quite blurred. In this situation the fastest aid is removing the aqueous with the canula. The silicone then enters the anterior chamber, comes in contact with the cornea and the fundus

123

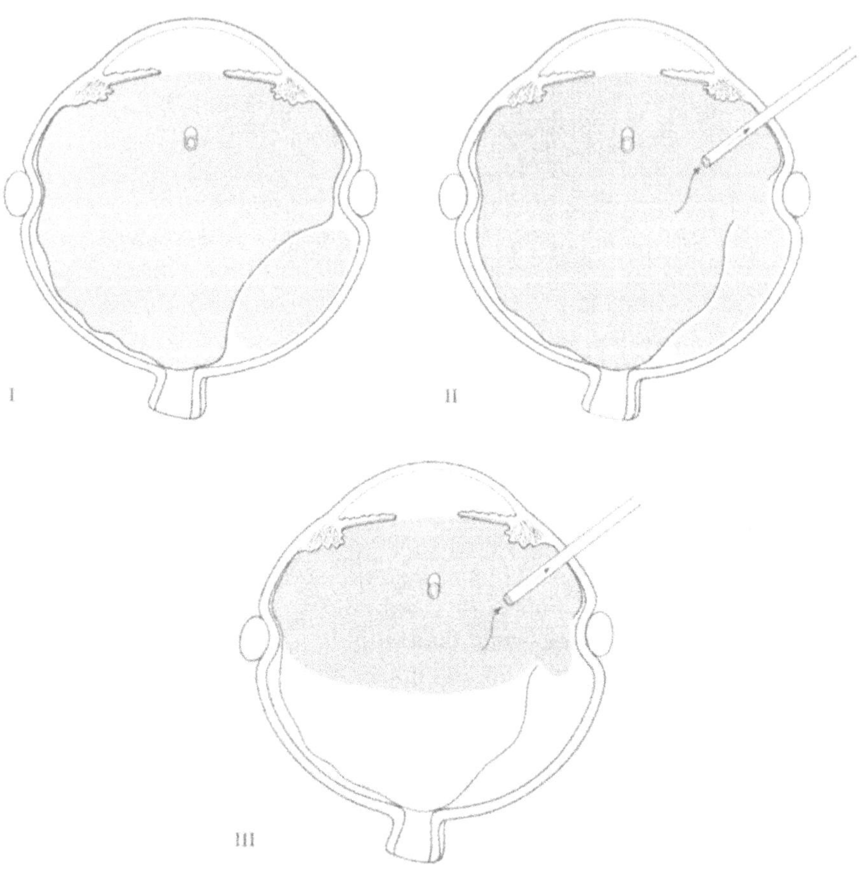

Figure 11. I, II, III. Removal of the large amount of silicone behind the retina. Through the large retinotomy the silicone behind the retina is joined with the big bubble and subsequently completely removed.

picture becomes sharp again. At the end of the operation the anterior chamber can be restored. With the low intraocular pressure some Ringer solution is injected through the iridectomy, by which the silicone bubble is pressed backward (Fig. 12 I, II, III, IV).

A particular optical problem is presented by intraocular lenses. Basically no IOL should be removed for optical reasons, yet they make the operation more difficult. The problem is the least with the iris fixed lenses which have become well adherent in the course of time. It is always possible to remove a part of the iris, respecting the fixed places, and to enlarge the pupil in this way. The posterior chamber lenses give the best view and the pupil can mostly be enlarged well. On the other hand, if the posterior capsula is very opaque, there is relatively little to be done, because the capsula serves as support for the lens

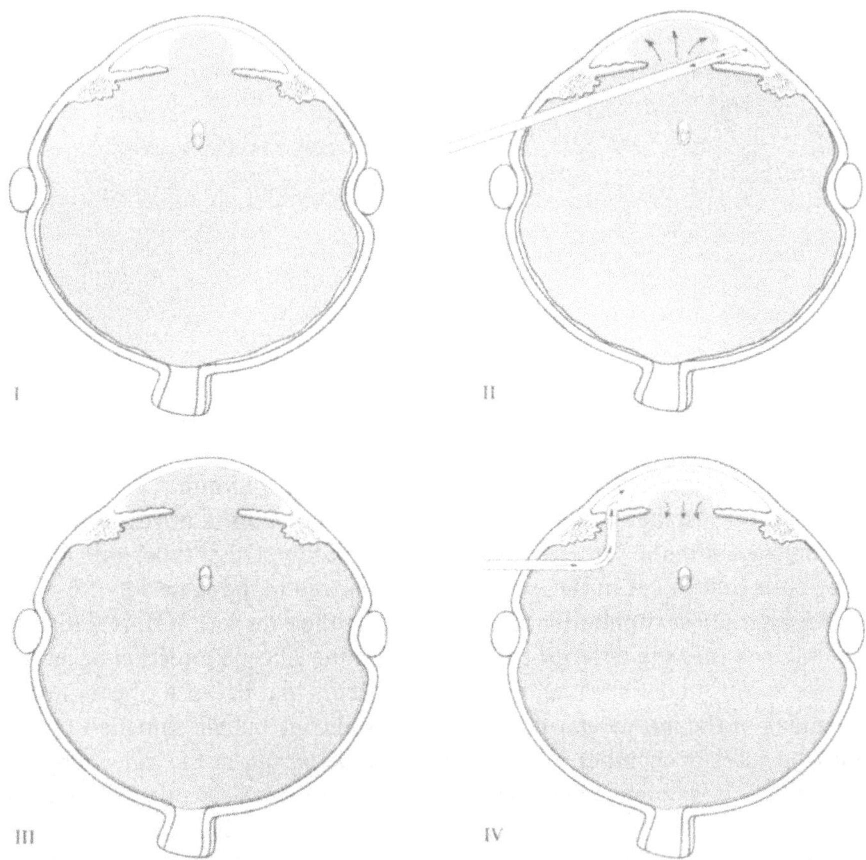

Figure 12. I: Prolapse of the silicone bubble through the pupil opening. Astigmatism and optical impediment; II: Evacuation of the aqueous – penetrating of the silicone into the anterior chamber; III: Improvement of optical situation by the good contact of the silicone with the cornea; IV: Restauration of the anterior chamber at the end of the operation.

and cannot be removed. In the most favourable situation it is possible to remove the posterior part of the capsula with the vitrectome if the lens is fixed in the periphery. With all lenses a 6 o'clock iridectomy should be performed to ensure staying of the silicone behind the diaphragm.

The greatest optical problem is the anterior chamber lenses because they are mostly fixed badly and because the pupil is often very narrow and not to be enlarged. With the wide pupil there is, with some types of the anterior chamber lenses (Choyce types), always the danger of luxation at the operation. For these reasons, in the eyes with the anterior chamber lense it is sometimes necessary to remove the lens. To avoid further operating with a fresh corneal wound we prefer removal of the lens through the enlarged pars

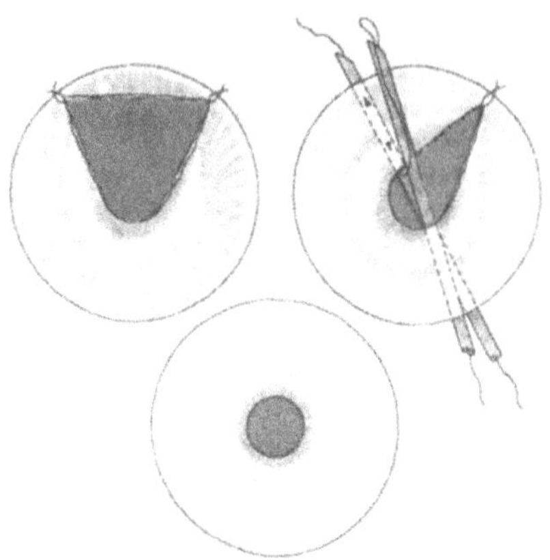

Figure 13. Temporary iris suture.

plana sclerotomy. The wound has to be enlarged to 7–8 mm. Closing of this sclerotomy is further without problems. Compact lenses (Choyce) can easily be removed with the forceps through the sclerotomy. Other types with plastic loops can first be cut in the eye and then removed in the same way.

An optically very disturbing complication in the eyes with IOL is getting of the silicone into the anterior chamber. After the silicone injection or during re-operations under silicone it sometimes occurs that because of continuous changing of the intraocular pressure a small silicone bubble somehow comes into the anterior chamber. As the opening in the capsula or the iridectomy are very small, it is practically impossible to press the small silicone bubble back through the hole to join the bubble behind the lens. The bubble has to be sucked out, but at the same time the Ringer solution has to be injected into the anterior chamber, because otherwise a new bubble presses into it. It is a very nerve-racking game, which is yet, mostly with a lot of patience, successful in the end. A preventing measure is injecting of Healon into the anterior chamber, which prevents getting of silicone into the anterior chamber.

The last peroperative complication that often threatens to make further operating practically impossible is the peroperative or also preoperative miosis. The solution we used to apply, the so-called surgical mydriasis, we have totally abandoned for the already mentioned reasons. Operating in the miosis in the aphakic eyes is possible but very difficult and time-consuming. Therefore we have taken enthusiastically Eckardt's idea of temporary iris suture. We have modified the technique a little, because we have found out that with two fixation sutures in the lower half one gets sufficiently enlarged pupil to work normally. The needle and the suture are the same we have described with the retinal suture (Fig. 13). In this way one gets a triangular pupil, which after the operation, without problems, becomes round again, perhaps a little enlarged.

126

7. Postoperative course I

Early postoperative complications

Already on the day following the operation the operated eyes are, as a rule, little irritated and painless. The reason is the silicone, which is not only inert but also exercising a stabilizing effect on the eye when injected in the optimum amount. Another reason is the absence of a severe operative trauma. The pre-existing buckles are not revised and setting of the encircling band in the first operations is little traumatizing. Immediately after the operation and also in the following days the patient does not need head positioning. On the first morning the anterior chamber is often flat due to the supine position of the patient after the operation. After getting up the aqueous will come into the anterior chamber through the 6 o'clock iridectomy and a normal depth will be restored.

After a long operation, particularly with a lot of retinal and anterior segment surgery, a fibrin reaction very frequently develops directly after the operation. On the first day a strong exudation in the anterior chamber can be observed, the iridectomy is mostly open and the fundus view not obscured. On the second day the fibrin mostly thickens into a clump and the anterior chamber becomes flat due to closing of the iridectomy. The fundus view becomes cloudy. This reaction can be very different in its intensity – from very thin membranes in the pupillary opening, which can hardly be observed without a slit lamp, to massive clumps which take 5 or 6 days to become reabsorbed. This reaction is mostly harmless, although it sometimes looks very impressive. Its consequences, though, can sometimes be unpleasant. As the first consequence one should mention closing of the 6 o'clock iridectomy. Sometimes the fibrin in the area of the iridectomy is not completely reabsorbed but slowly organized, by which a fibrotic membrane develops which blocks the iridectomy. At an early stage of development this membrane can be easily destroyed by YAG or Argon laser. The same treatment later, when the membrane has become fibrotic and the iris shrunken, is little successful, because it is often accompanied by haemorrhages which stimulate the development of new membranes. A surgical iridectomy is to be preferred to laser treatment in this case.

A second disturbing consequence of incomplete reabsorption of the fibrin develops in the eyes with intraocular lenses. A thin membrane remains on the front surface of the lens, which can significantly disturb the fundus view. A non-invasive therapy after development of the membrane is not possible.

The fibrin reaction is a complication that, although it mostly disappears spontaneously, certainly has to be treated for these reasons. We are not convinced of advantages of oral therapy with corticosteroids and we are satisfied with intensive local therapy. This therapy has its full effect in most cases. It has yet to be mentioned that these complications cause no subjective complaints to the patients. If they are not accompanied by increase of pressure, the patient has no pain, and clouding of light at the early postoperative stage does not strike the patient. Absence of pain is one of the most important symptoms that distinguish the fibrin reaction at the earliest stage from the bacterial endophthalmitis.

In our experience of nearly nine years with far more than a thousand operations we have seen only four cases of postoperative endophthalmitis. As it concerns few cases that had an unusual course it seems to us worth closer examining.

The first case developed endophthalmitis after the second operation. It concerned an eye with a nearly total traumatic aniridia and aphakia. The eye was entirely filled with silicone, the cornea was in contact with silicone and the anterior chamber did not exist. Therefore the symptoms of the anterior segment, such as clouding of the cornea and hypopyon or exudation into the anterior chamber, were, as not possible, absent. In spite of subjective complaints of the patient the diagnosis was not established, and only when after a few days the accumulation of pus was seen in the inferior part behind the silicone bubble was the situation recognized. As the function, which had been poor before, practically completely disappeared in the meantime, and as the second eye was concerned, the patient was not operated on, but was treated conservatively. With this therapy the eye was preserved, without function.

The second patient had subjective complaints. It was a case operated twice, with total detachment and PVR. The subjective symptoms appeared a few days after the surgery. The eye had a lens, symptoms in the anterior segment were not alarming and the fundus view was not obscured. After 2 days one could first see, with the contact glass, a pussy exudation in the temporal and inferior part behind the lens and in front of the silicone bubble, which expanded very thinly behind the silicone. The patient was operated on the next day. The silicone and the lens were removed, pussy infiltrations were found in the area of the infusion sclerotomy. After the repeated vitrectomy and rinsing with an antibiotic, silicone was injected again. The situation of the retina about a week after the latest operation naturally did not allow removal of silicone. The eye and the function were rescued.

The last two cases were aphakic with the silicone bubble behind the diaphragm and developed the symptoms on the second day after surgery. In both cases there were subjective complaints together with appearance of strong exudation with hypopyon in the anterior chamber. As the cornea was clear, the fundus view was little disturbed. Both patients were operated on the same day. Removal of silicone with rinsing of the eye with antibiotic was performed. A clear localization of the beginning of the process could not be proved. At the end of the operation silicone was injected again. One eye was rescued including the function, the other, after the initial success, developed a redetachment after a few days and because of the bad function, as the second eye, it was not reoperated.

With the description of these cases we wanted to point out that endophthalmitis due to presence of silicone in the eye frequently shows different symptoms and sometimes developes slowlier. Prompt operating immediately following recognition of the first symptoms is indicated. Re-injection of silicone at the end of the operation in these eyes, in which no stable situation has been achieved in the posterior segment, is an absolute necessity.

Haemorrhages in the anterior chamber secondary to the operation are extremely rare. Mostly it concerns haemorrhages from the area of the 6 o'clock iridectomy. The consequence is sometimes closing and not functioning of the iridectomy after reabsorption. This unnecessary complication is completely avoidable with a good haemostasis of the iridectomy site. Haemorrhages in the posterior segment are avoidable for the greatest part, at least in the PVR and trauma cases. These haemorrhages, which are not very massive, are to be seen after endocryopexy and occur much less frequently after endolaser coagulation. They are hardly ever so massive that they have to be evacuated and mostly gradually reabsorb spontaneously. We are convinced, though, that they play their own part in development of reproliferations. To avoid this complication is, then, also the best that can be done. In diabetic traction detachments the situation is somewhat different. It is certain that also here very much can be prevented by careful diathermocoagulation, yet sometimes (especially in bad young cases) massive secondary haemorrhages occur after the operation. The next day massive haemorrhage is to be seen behind the silicone bubble, which, due to its volume presses the silicone bubble forwards and in this way moves the whole diaphragm forwards. Apart from these disturbed relations in the anterior segment, by which intraocular pressure can raise as well, such a haemorrhage is a very serious postoperative complication, and the blood ought to be removed as soon as possible (within a few days). With the diabetics this blood reabsorbs very slowly or not at all and represents feeding ground for new proliferations.

Postoperative increase of intraocular pressure is no rarity. It develops mostly on the second postoperative day and has two different causes. The first is development of a kind of 'ghost cells glaucoma' after the extensive operation. In these cases silicone is behind the diaphragm, the iridectomy is open and the anterior chamber is normally deep. Increasing of pressure probably develops due to blocking of the trabecular system by cells and waste products that float in the chamber aqueous. The pressure level is mostly moderate, between 20 and 30 mm, and the patient does not have too many complaints. The corneal epithelium can be a little cloudy and the fundus view is disturbed. The pressure reacts well to drug therapy, but this should be applied only in case of subjective complaints. The pressure, namely, often normalizes spontaneously and the eye can tolerate it without damage for a few days.

The second cause is purely mechanical and occurs because silicone, for one or the other reason, has penetrated forwards or even into the anterior chamber. To understand this mechanism better, the significance and working of the 6 o'clock iridectomy should be discussed first.

In vitrectomized aphakic eyes the silicone bubble floats freely in the posterior segment and is in a close or loose contact with the iris, depending on its size and position. If overfilling occurs, the bubble is too big for the volume of the posterior segment, it presses the diaphragm forward with its mass and prolapses more or less through the pupil into the anterior segment. The same situation can also develop with smaller bubbles in certain circumstances with the optimum filling. Such a bubble is in a loose contact with the iris and the aqueous can basically flow through the pupil from the posterior to the anterior chamber in the perpendicular head position. That will occur more easily with the wide than with the narrow pupil, but it will be quite impossible in the lying position of the head. In this position the floating silicone bubble will completely block the pupil and the aqueous will flow backward, behind the bubble, being heavier than silicone. Change of the head position will not help any more after some time, when enough aqueous has accumulated behind the bubble and the bubble is pressed upward and forward. In this way a complete pupillary block gradually develops, because more and more produced aqueous accumulates at the back and the bubble presses the diaphragm more and more forward. In the end it will depend on the absorption speed of the enclosed aqueous in the anterior chamber whether silicone will fill the whole anterior chamber or slowly close the chamber angle and press the whole iris against the cornea. The final result is the same: very high intraocular pressure, first due to the pupillary block and finally due to the chamber angle block. The intraocular pressure will once be increased because of filling of the anterior chamber with silicone, another time because of shifting of the diaphragm and complete closing of the angle.

Due to this mechanism two very important complications can develop in the silicone surgery. In the extreme cases a medically untreatable malignant glaucoma develops, in which the surgical intervention is the only, fortunately successful, solution. In the cases in which this mechanism functions only partly, a contact of the silicone bubble with the cornea develops leading to corneopathy. This situation is again (depending on the aqueous production and a few other factors) frequently combined with the chronic glaucoma due to the incomplete pupillary block.

This mechanism, known for years as the malignant glaucoma in the glaucoma surgery, has caused a lot of complications in this surgery for years and has influenced the final result negatively in many cases. Our accepting of all these complication as granted for many years and our unquestioning dedication to their arduous and often unsuccessful treatment, testifies to professional blindness occurring time and again.

Deliverance came through introduction of the 6 o'clock iridectomy by Ando. This little intervention was simple and logical and established communication between the two eye chambers. The aqueous could in this way flow into the anterior chamber, accumulation of the aqueous behind the silicone bubble was prevented and at the same time cohesion forces of silicone made the bubble stay behind the diaphragm (Fig. 1 I, II, III, IV).

The technical performance of iridectomy is simple and has already been described. There are two more remarks to be done. During the performing of iridectomy no tissue remnants (lens, capsula, scars) must be left behind the iris – they have to be removed first, and the iridectomy has to be large. Both mentioned points are of basic importance for functioning of the iridectomy.

It is not exaggerated to say that introduction of the 6 o'clock iridectomy has revolutionized this surgery. Owing to it not only was the contact of silicone with the cornea avoided and glaucoma prevented, but also early surgery of the lens was made possible. The patient has been spared many operations and the final results have also been improved.

Development of high intraocular pressure after the operation is better comprehensible through understanding of the described mechanisms. Clinically two causes can be stated, basically mechanical ones. The first is not functioning of iridectomy, mostly due to blood or fibrin clots in the iridectomy opening, the second is overfilling of silicone. In the first situation the best solution is waiting and local treatment with corticosteroids (as described under the fibrin reaction). When the pressure is too high the iridectomy has to be opened with the laser or surgically. In the second situation, the prevention is the best that can be done. When once occurred, there is no use waiting. Silicone mostly fills the whole anterior chamber, the iridectomy is sometimes even open but blocked from both sides by silicone. If in this situation iridectomy is not open either and is covered by a membrane, subsequent opening with the laser has no effect, because silicone is closing the iridectomy from

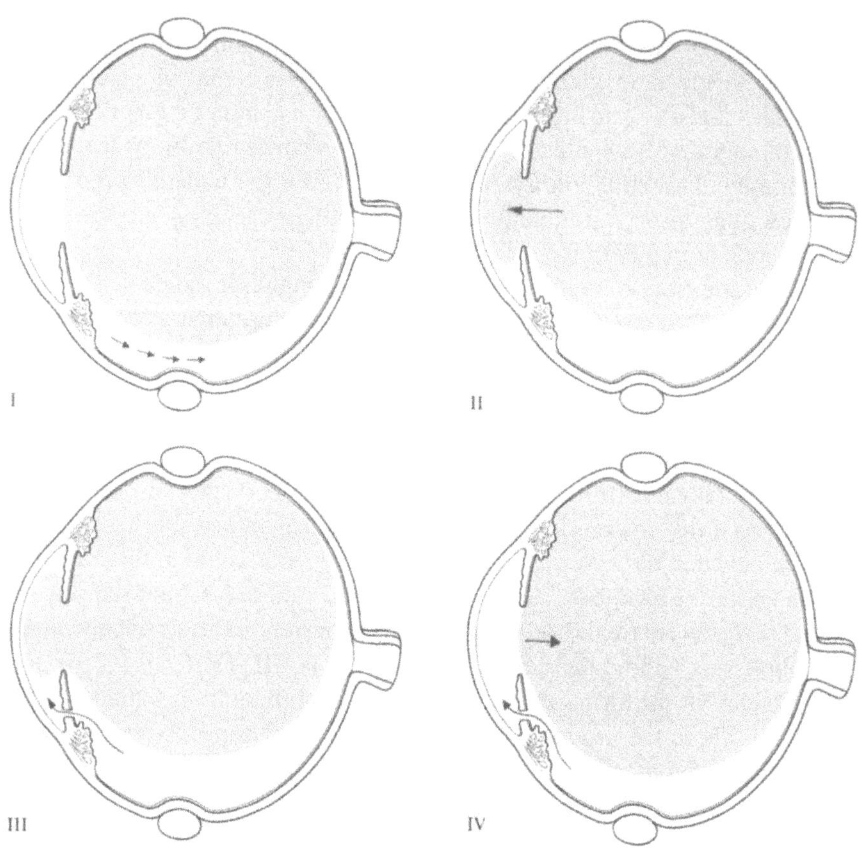

Figure 1. I, II. Accumulation of the aqueous behind the silicone bubble and penetration of the silicone into the anterior chamber – development of the pupillary block; III, & IV: Through the 6 o'clock iridectomy the communication between the posterior and anterior chamber is restored and the silicone bubble is pushed backward.

both sides. The only solution is to open the eye – best corneally, to release some silicone and to fill the anterior chamber with the Ringer solution.

This complication mostly starts developing already during the operation. The eye is filled with too much silicone, the iridectomy is indeed open but blocked directly from behind by silicone. The produced aqueous, because of closed iridectomy, gets immediately backwards. Horizontal head position even deteriorates the situation. When the aqueous is absorbed in the anterior chamber, the situation is completely bad, because then the silicone bubble pushed from backward fills up the anterior chamber.

This complication can be completely avoided if at the end of the operation, the anterior chamber is filled with water at least so far that the iridectomy is free from silicone. During this filling of the anterior chamber the intraocular pressure has to be very low. Otherwise the injected fluid will immediately get backward behind the silicone bubble. Subsequently silicone can be carefully injected until the intraocular pressure has been normalized.

As the last early complication one should mention penetrating of the isolated silicone bubble into the anterior chamber. At the early stage of our surgery it occurred more frequently and meant that during the surgery one had broken the zonula because of the increased intraocular pressure, which as a consequence made penetration of the isolated silicone bubble into the anterior chamber possible. Since we have nearly always removed the lens during the first operation, this complication has become correspondingly more rare and still occurs practically only with the IOL. The mechanism is the same, particularly with the posterior chamber lenses with which the posterior capsula and zonula are still intact. On the first day after the surgery small or bigger silicone bubbles are seen floating in the anterior chamber. This occurs much more frequently after an operation during which the same difficulties with intruding of silicone were encountered. Although the bubble has been removed from the anterior chamber in the already described way, it is to be found there again the next day. This complication is not serious because such a mobile silicone bubble does not mean danger for the cornea and only exceptionally should be removed at an early stage. It is best to wait until silicone can be removed or another operation is necessary for any reason (reproliferation).

Late postoperative complications

Late complications following vitrectomy combined with silicone injection consist for the greatest part of three groups. These are the complications concerning the cornea, the lens and the complications developed through emulsification of silicone oil. The complications concerning the retina are for the greatest part due to persistence of the proliferative process and should be described separately.

Problems with the cornea develop exclusively because of the permanent contact of silicone with the cornea endothelium and since the introduction of the 6 o'clock iridectomy have become rare. As the first symptom the band-shaped keratopathy should be mentioned. It develops in eyes in which the greatest part of the cornea has been in permanent contact with silicone. First symptoms appear after three till six months. It concerns the calcium salt deposits in Bowman's layer and superficial stroma. Once started, the changes will increase relatively fast and opacify a wide zone of the cornea completely. These changes can be explained by blocking of endothelium and subsequent deficient nutrition of the cornea, especially of the superficial layers. Strongly decreased circulation of the aqueous in these eyes probably plays a role as well. Even before these changes appear, thinning of the corneal stroma can be observed, which is detactable pachometrically. It is also to be explained with the endothelium block induced by silicone oil. The corneal endothelium is not only disturbed in its function through the contact with silicone, but also, if the contact has been long enough, irreversibly damaged. This damage starts after a few months, but unfortunately, as long as the silicone is in contact with the endothelium, it is not detectable clinically and photographically. The refractive index of silicone and the corneal stroma are, namely, nearly the same, which makes biomicroscopy and photography of the endothelium with the specular microscope impossible. The changes of the endothelium reach from severe damage of the endothelium cells to metaplasia and formation of a new collagen layer. This transformation of the endothelium together with the fact that, certainly at the early stage, it is difficult or impossible to recognize it in the given situation, has a great clinical significance.

The described complications should not occur any more in the eyes with the preserved diaphragm. With an optimum silicone filling and open iridectomy we have never seen the silicone in the anterior chamber. Yet there are still patients in whom there is no iris present and in whom the contact with the silicone is unavoidable. The patients who have been followed-up badly and appear after a long time with closed iridectomy, corneopathy and high IOP are another, unfortunately rather large group that has to be treated for these complications.

The most logical treatment is breaking of the contact between the cornea and the silicone by removing of the silicone or pressing the silicone back behind the diaphragm. Removing of the silicone will completely depend on the situation in the posterior segment, which is possible to estimate before the operation. What is not to be estimated is the situation of the endothelium and the consequences that removal of the silicone will have for the cornea. As we have mentioned before, the situation of the endothelium before the operation is not to be judged. The corneal stroma is, due to the endothelium block by the silicone, completely transparent before the operation. It will, though, if the endothelium is damaged, become totally opaque after removal of the silicone, because the damaged endothelium offers no more protection against invasion of the aqueous.

At the late stage of endothelial damage, in which a retrocorneal collagen membrane has developed, the cornea decompensation will not occur because the newly developed membrane offers enough protection against invasion of the aqueous. The transparence of the cornea, though, leaves a lot to be desired in these cases.

On the other side of the cornea the calcium salt deposits are easy to remove with EDTA-Na solution after an epithelium abrasion. However, this presents the final solution only if afterwards the silicone is not in contact with the endothelium any more.

134

In the treatment of silicone corneopathy all these facts have to be taken into account. In the early cases the removal of the silicone or pressing of the silicone bubble backward, combined with 'cleaning' of the cornea with the EDTA-Na solution, will bring the desired result. It is often surprising how clean the cornea can become after this treatment. In the cases in which the endothelium is severely damaged, the perforating keratoplasty remains as the only good solution. Unfortunately, there will always remain enough cases in which, for various reasons, the removal of silicone during keratoplasty is not possible. In these cases the keratoplasty is a palliative solution, because in a few months the transplant will become opaque again in the same way and repeating of the same operation will be necessary.

It remains to be remarked that with the advanced corneal opacities before the removal of silicone the patient should be informed about the possibility of corneal decompensation. A perforating keratoplasty a few days afterwards should best be already planned as a precaution.

Development of cataract after the operation was an almost unavoidable complication before the introduction of the 6 o'clock iridectomy. Opacity of the lens had, in our opinion, not so much to do with the silicone but much more with the proliferative process itself and with the surgical treatment notwithstanding whether it was performed with or without silicone.

In the eyes which used to be operated in the original J. Scott's technique and in which the silicone was mostly not in contact with the lens, cataract did not develop slowlier and not faster either than in the eyes that were vitrectomized. With such a great variety of cases, not only as far as pathology is concerned, but also concerning preoperative course, number of operations and course of the last operation, it is very difficult to say why the cataract developed. For us it was never a question of practical importance either, as we always thought that development of cataract was for the greatest part unavoidable. Since we decided to remove the lens in the first operation, this problem has lost importance even further. Apart from this, the problem of cataract treatment of the earlier operated patients will remain. Therefore this problem seems to us worth examining.

There is not much to be reported on the time of development of cataract and its form, as they differ from case to case. In younger patients cataract sometimes developed very fast after the lens had stayed clear for a long time after the operation. Due to fast swelling of the lens acute pressure rises occurred so that the lens had to be removed quickly. In older patients the slow development was rather characteristic.

In the cataract surgery the choice of operative treatment depended always on whether or not to remove the silicone. In the first years mostly not vitrectomized eyes were concerned and removal of the silicone together with the cataract extraction was seldom possible. Therefore the extracapsular technique was chosen, which with soft lenses was carried out in an irigation-aspiration procedure while with hard lenses one operated ab externo. The experience with extracapsular extraction was very negative because shortly after the operation a massive secondary cataract developed, which obstructed the visus and the fundus view very much. In the cases in which the silicone was to be removed during the same operation one operated intracapsularly, either through the pars plana or ab externo.

After the negative experience with the extracapsular surgery one stepped over to the intracapsular technique. One used Healon with the extraction to avoid leaking out of silicone, which proved as good in a great number of cases. With the introduction of the 6 o'clock iridectomy the whole problem of cataract extraction became much simpler because pressing of silicone into the anterior chamber did not represent a problem any more.

In the present surgery the intracapsular technique is always chosen because we think that the capsular remnants, particularly when the silicone is left in the eye, represent a provocation or at least a scaffolding for the proliferative process. We have never performed simultaneous removal of the silicone and the extracapsular cataract extraction and implantation of a posterior chamber lens and we think that this is a daring operation. It should not, though, be basically rejected and should perhaps be left for selected cases (diabetics?).

Basically, one tries to remove the lens through the pars plana. The eye is connected to the infusion without letting it flow. As the eye is filled with silicone another infusion cannula with liquid is introduced through one of the sclerotomies into the lens. Through another sclerotomy the vitrectome is introduced and the lens mass in the capsula removed in this way. Removal of the capsula with the forceps follows, because the silicone already appears in the pupil opening at this moment. After removal of the capsula the fundus is inspected and if there are no objections to removing of the silicone the first infusion is opened and the silicone removed from the eye under controlled pressure. If during the inspection one detects that for whatever reason the silicone should be left in the eye, a 6 o'clock iridectomy is performed and the eye connected to the silicone infusion. According to the existing situation one can, if necessary, either operate in the posterior segment or only fill up the eye with silicone.

The same technique can also be followed with hard lenses, which have to be operated transcorneally. After removal of the lens and a position suture of the cornea, the fundus can be inspected through the contact lens. The disadvantage is that the pupil often becomes very narrow after the cataract extraction and makes the fundus view difficult. The silicone can then be evacuated through the corneal wound, after removal of the position suture or in another case, if necessary, after preparing the iridectomy the eye can be filled up with silicone.

136

The described complications are consequences of a mechanical interaction between the tissue and silicone. It is certainly true for changes of the cornea, much less for cataract, which is also caused by the basic disease. Complications caused by emulsification of silicone are, however, consequences of physico-chemical properties of silicone. Emulsification means development of small silicone bubbles or particles, which in certain circumstances get loose from the big silicone bubble and move freely in the remaining space. The latest investigations show that the property to develop emulsification is different with various kinds of silicone, and among other things depends on molecular weight of silicone molecules. The silicones with molecules with low molecular weight or the silicones that are not completely pure and contain a strong component of such molecules should emulsify faster and easier. It seems to us, that besides these physico-chemical properties, which are certainly very important, the mechanical component is of a great importance as well. In our opinion, it is exactly the mechanical component that provokes emulsification, which is, again, generated more easily or more difficult in various kinds of silicone. We base this assertion on clinical experience, which has often shown that with a smaller silicone bubble that floats free and mobile in the eye, the first signs of emulsification appear very soon.

In the eyes which were operated in the 60s, when one injected silicone in the vitreal space without a good optical control and therefore in small amounts (1–2 ml) following only drainage of subretinal fluid, one noticed that the silicone emulsified very soon and entered the anterior chamber already after a few days. On the other hand, the eyes operated in the original Scott's technique, in which under optical control after drainage of the subretinal fluid and evacuation of the fluid vitreous and the simultaneous silicone injection, the whole intravitreal space is filled with silicone, such eyes often do not show any signs of emulsification even after many years. In these eyes, in the ideal case, the silicone bubble is posteriorly in contact with the attached retina, anteriorly separated from the anterior segment by the residual vitreous and proliferative membranes, and practically encapsulated in this way. Further contraction of the membranes around the silicone bubble, which progresses after the operation due to persisting of the proliferative process, only reinforces this capsula and immobilizes the silicone bubble entirely. It is noticeable with operating of such eyes (removal of silicone, vitrectomy) how little emulsified silicone is to be found behind the membranes and that the fibrotic membranes around the silicone bubble have completely substituted the formed vitreous.

Another situation develops in the eyes which were operated in the last years. Due to radical vitrectomy, by which all fibrotic structures are removed, a space develops in which only the iris diaphragm separates the silicone bubble from the anterior chamber. As we know, an ideal contact of the silicone with the surrounding structures is not possible, because there is always a water layer between them. Owing to elasticity of the iris, even with the optimum filling, constant movement of the silicone bubble in the eye is unavoidable. The result is appearance of emulsified silicone in the anterior chamber sooner or later, depending on filling of the eye. In our patients it takes on average 3–6 months until the first symptoms can be observed. Due to expansion of the small silicone bubble after some time an accumulation develops in the upper part of the anterior chamber with the level downwards. In the eyes in which the big bubble does not completely fill the posterior segment, one can see the emulsified silicone with the typical level also behind the bubble. This extreme picture is rather rare and develops relatively slowly.

In the eyes which function normally and have not the low or too high intraocular pressure, the small silicone bubbles are taken away with the aqueous and certain balance develops between the produced emulsion and outflow of the anterior chamber. This balance will not last long and will gradually pass into the increase of intraocular pressure. Probably it concerns a slow obstruction of the trabecular meshwork by sedimentation of small silicone bubbles. Another extreme is the eyes with a very low intraocular pressure. These eyes have practically no aqueous production and small or very low outflow, and without silicone could not function at all. In these eyes a permanent emulsification can be observed through which very remarkable clinical pictures develop without intraocular pressure being changed at all.

The tiny silicone bubbles in the aqueous as the first symptom of emulsification are in a small amount still not a danger signal and not a reason for removal of silicone. Yet a regular control of the pressure in intervals of a few weeks is certainly indicated in this situation. If the increase of emulsification is accompanied with the rise of intraocular pressure, removal of silicone is necessary. The removal of silicone should be performed before development of glaucoma. The experience teaches that in spite of the removal of silicone normalizing of the intraocular pressure after that cannot be taken for granted. Medical therapy of glaucoma before and after removal of silicone is possible. Most eyes react very well on the production reducing drugs as well as on the miotics, and surgical treatment has very seldom been necessary by now.

However, we are far from underestimating these complications. In contrast to corneal changes and cataract, which are very limited owing to new developments in surgery, the development of glaucoma subsequent to emulsification of silicone, just because of development of our surgical concept and its radicality, has become an increasing problem. Use of purified silicone to diminish emulsification will probably somewhat postpone the development of this problem, but not prevent it. Early removal of silicone is the best solution, but it depends on the situation of the retina and the dynamics of the proliferative process itself.

The complications we have described by now, like corneal changes and glaucoma, are totally or, like cataract, only partly a consequence of presence of silicone in the eye. It is common to all these complications that they, although different, have developed in the mechanical way and they can be explained so theoretically and clinically. Due to improved surgical technique and perhaps due to use of purified silicone these complications are avoidable to a certain degree and if once started they are also manageable.

The question whether silicone, besides the described, mechanically caused complications, also has some other effects in the eye, is difficult to answer. In general this question can be answered neither affirmatively nor negatively, because it does not concern a standardized product. In a certain degree this fact already devaluates all proofs from the past that tried to prove toxicity of silicone, simply because it was not always clear which silicone was concerned.

With the remark that we speak only about the silicone that we have used in our surgical activity for several years, we can say that we have found no proofs for toxical activity of silicone. As the other authors, we have also seen that electrophysiological examinations in the eyes filled with silicone have no diagnostic value. Because of insulating property of silicone these results are negative, after removal of silicone the values rise up to the limits which correspond to the situation of the retina. The pathoanatomic findings published on different sides as well as with us are certainly not to be minimized although they have mostly been done in enucleated eyes damaged by various factors. In which way the little silicone bubbles get into the tissue and evoke inflammatory reactions there is not completely clear. As there are indications which point that this process occurs more with the detached retina than with the normal, it would suggest that rather a biological process (macrophage?) is concerned than an active physical property of silicone. Penetrating of the small silicone bubble into the other tissue (e.g. opticus) was also observed in the enucleated eyes that had suffered under high intraocular pressure for a long time. It is possible that there are different ways in which silicone gets into the tissue and causes a reaction there. This reaction, though, is more of an inflammatory than chemotoxical kind. It is certainly so that toxical reactions are possible too in the use of certain silicone oils, but they are probably caused by the other elements in a not purified silicone. To ascribe these complications unconditionally to silicone will not bring the discussion about this, already complicated enough theme, any further.

In the everyday clinical work we could find no indications either which could point to the toxical activity of silicone. Pathoanatomical changes were comprehensible in almost all eyes and could be related either to the described complications and their mechanisms or to the preceding damages of the eye. One of these changes is the late starting and slowly progressing opticus atrophy. There, deterioration of visual field does not run parallelly to the clinical picture at all, on the contrary, the visual field remains unchanged for a long time. In the last time we analyzed a great number of patients and, although it concerned the cases difficult to compare, we stated that nearly always the eyes were concerned which had been severely damaged before surgery and for that reason too needed several operations with extreme surgery. Among the eyes there were conspicuously many cases with perforating wounds and severe damages with the trauma, which after silicone injection still were very hypotonic. These are the eyes still functioning at the edge of atrophy and certainly not able to exist without silicone. On the contrary, a lot of our patients, who have been operated successfully, show no complications and tolerate silicone without any secondary changes for 7–8 years. They are mostly patients operated in original Scott's technique who have not developed any emulsification. The reason that silicone has not been removed from these eyes after so many years is simply that these patients have no complaints whatsoever and refuse a new operation for removal of silicone.

8. Postoperative course II

Persistance of PVR

Persisting of the proliferative process after the operation remains the main problem in vitreoretinal surgery. This problem burdens in a negative sense the final results of the surgery much more than all complications developed by or without silicone.

The reason for persisting of proliferative processes, often called reproliferations, is to be sought in a combination of all already described factors and in the surgical intervention itself. It is certainly so that by the operation a great part of the factors important for the proliferative process as pathophysiological stimulances (hypotony, exudates, inflammation, etc.) are removed together with mechanical factors (traction, scars, membranes), but it is also certain that all stimulating factors cannot be removed in any case. The surgical procedure applied to alter this complicated pathoanatomical situation has beside positive effects some negative consequences as well. It is unavoidable that after the operation, however atraumatically one may work, beside tissue damages also debris, blood and tissue remnants are left in the eye. Under circumstances, these can also have a stimulating effect on reproliferations.

As the third factor the time of the operation should be mentioned. Although the proliferative process can nearly always be found in the eye at various stages, the removal of the proliferative tissue is particularly difficult at an early stage, at which the fibrosing has not yet occurred. Consequently, the reproliferation in early operated eyes is to be expected much more frequently than in the eyes with the long-existing PVR, in which most fibrotic structures are easier to remove. Beside all these factors, which again have not an absolute value for the development of reproliferations, the primary disease is also of great importance for the postoperative course.

It can be understood from this discussion that even the most correctly performed operation offers no guarantee against development of reproliferations. Yet it is plausible that with an operation performed less correctly and especially with disregarding of certain rules and basic principles, the chance of failure through development of reproliferations is significantly greater. Therefore, in the following description of the manifestation of reproliferations and their treatment we shall concentrate on description of reproliferations following an operation with a so-called normal course. At the end we shall mention in a few words the complications developed after badly performed operations.

Although it has no practical significance any more, it still seems important to us in order to understand the process of reproliferations to describe their manifestation in the patients operated in the original Scott's technique first. As described already, in these patients, as they had not been vitrectomized, nearly always after the operation a residual detachment was left anterior to the buckle. After a few days or weeks a redetachment sometimes developed in the inferior part in the eyes with centrally attached retina. The reason was twofold. Due to further circular contraction of the peripheral proliferative membranes, frequently connected to the vitreous base, the existing peripheral detachment increased and spread out centrally over the buckle. The second reason was the epiretinal proliferation central to the buckle, which slowly raised the retina, sometimes spread out over the buckle to the periphery and joined the existing peripheral detachment. Frequently both mechanisms were combined. The rhegmatogenous element, if ever, appeared only later mostly owing to traction induced opening of previous peripheral holes, and worsened the developed situation. In the greatest number of cases this situation occurred in the inferior part and therefore gave rise to different interpretations and therapeutic measures. Without entering into the particulars of each of them it does seem useful to us to express our opinion on this problem.

First, if we analyze this problem in various indication groups, we shall see that it exists as such only with idiopathic retinal detachments with PVR and in a smaller amount with giant tears. With traumatic retinal detachments with PVR localisation of redetachment frequently depends on the perforation wound. With reproliferations and redetachments of the diabetic traction detachment this problem does not appear at all.

Analyzing further the largest group, the idiopathic retinal detachments with PVR, we want to mention that preceding the conventional surgery in the greatest number of cases the pathology (retinal tears) having caused the detachment is concentrated in the superior quadrants. Correspondingly, the therapeutic measures are also emphatically applied in the superior quadrants. This results in scarring of the greatest part of the periphery with complete or incomplete closing of holes. The postoperative development of PVR may occur due to incomplete closing of holes or in spite of complete closing of holes, because the proliferative process has already progressed so far and is not to be stopped any more by excluding the rhegmatogenic factor. Initially the development is slow and accompanied or jointly provoked by accumulation of subretinal fluid in inferior quandrants. Simultaneously we can observe sedimentation of pigment cells on the retinal surface in the inferior quadrants, which occurs there for obvious reasons of gravitation. The following stage is the development of starfolds and the increase of detachment, which frequently spreads out slightly over the circular buckle, as there are few or no retinopexy scars. The final result is the well-known picture of PVR detachment with domineering changes and the epicentre in the inferior periphery. In the cases that were first operated successfully the PVR detachment develops relatively suddenly, but already before its development the signs of infiltration of the vitreous with pigment cells are noticeable together with reduced vitreous mobility and, which is particularly important, sedimentation of pigment cells on the surface of the inferior retina (gravitation reasons). The detachment develops when the membranes have reached a certain degree of maturity and start contracting. Here again it is to be seen that most pathological changes and the epicentre of starfolds are concentrated in the inferior part. Deviating developments can be seen in the cases in which for various reasons during the conventional surgery haemorrhages, perforations with or without retina incarceration or overtreatment of cryocoagulation occurred. There the proliferative process begins at the corresponding site and spreads out further. These are, however, exceptional situations, which resemble more to the development following traumas.

If we keep in mind this development of the proliferative process, we can also understand why after vitrectomy combined with silicone oil injection in this group problems began again there where they were to be found most frequently and where they were most difficult to deal with. Reproliferation after the operation begins again most often in the inferior central part of the retina because there proliferative changes are strongest and because during the surgery there were unavoidably most iatrogenic damages. The entire process is also stimulated by the fact that after the operation all sorts of debris, blood and cells accumulate in the inferior part for gravitation reasons. The reduced circulation of fluid behind the silicone bubble and the reduced space become yet additional factors for development of the proliferative process. The fact that the mechanical tamponade of the silicone bubble in the inferior part, by the physical property of silicone, has little or no effect, may also play a role, but not a major one, in the entire complex process. The rhegmatogenous factor (the open and leaking retinal hole), so often suspected as the cause of detachment, plays in this connection hardly ever a decisive role in the correctly performed operation. The best proof for this is that in the correctly and successfully operated cases the first signs of retinal detachment occur only after a few days. The cause of the detachment, if not evident in the first days yet always within a short time, is the traction of proliferative membranes. Opening of the already existing holes or tearing of new ones develops mostly secondarily and complicates the whole situation in a certain degree.

The whole process develops in case of giant tears in a similar way. A special feature regarding giant tears is the frequent development of a macula pucker in the postoperative course, which very often is not accompanied by the development of detachment.

In traumatic cases the postoperative development of reproliferations is less typical and highly dependent on the intensity and form of the perforating injury itself. Beside all the above-mentioned factors the greatest source of complications is the perforation scar. This relates in particular to the chorioretinal scars in the posterior segment, which are still active after a very long time.

Since we realized that the main source of reproliferations in diabetic traction detachment are the residual tissue remnants of the fibrovascular membranes, and since we remove them very carefully during the operation, the number of redetachments in diabetic cases has strongly decreased. Reproliferations in diabetic traction detachment are, in biological as well as in clinical sense, not strictly the same processes as in PVR detachments and therefore the pathoanatomical picture differs from the above described groups. The main sources of reproliferations are secondary haemorrhages and probably the sites of previous vitreoretinal adhesions, and sometimes also the edges of iatrogenic holes or retinectomies. As the primary changes were concentrated in the posterior pole, the beginnings of reproliferations are also mostly to be found first in the centre. Our experience is that diabetic cases are, compared to the other groups, best to be kept under control concerning reproliferations. With careful removal of fibrovascular membranes and very accurate coagulation of bleeding spots after the silicone injection, the development of reproliferations in diabetic traction detachments can be prevented in the greatest number of cases.

In the past, in course of years, the described development of reproliferations was for us the main reason to change the original surgical technique and to develop the present surgical conception. Already in the beginning we realized that the unsolved problem of the peripheral residual detachment was a great source of postoperative complications. To eliminate this source we began to remove the vitreous and the other structures in the periphery as radically as possible. Since we have been doing this, the problems with traction from the periphery on the central retina, with correctly performed surgery, have practically disappeared. How much we have moved the problems more centrally and closer to the ciliary body owing to use of this radical surgery remains, naturally, without answer, but it is certain that we have significantly improved our results with clearing of the periphery. The main problems in all groups concentrate now, even if different from group to group, on the proliferation in the posterior pole, centrally from the buckle.

144

There is, though, a very small number of cases which represent an exception in the great number of operated patients and also an unsolvable problem for the time being. They are nearly without exception patients with perforating injuries, in whom the perforation site was in the anterior part of the eye and in whom the ciliary body was damaged at the time of injury or due to development thereafter. The preoperative hypotony has hardly been improved by the operation and although the posterior segment looks good and the retina is attached, a slowly progressing bulbus atrophy is to be observed. Improved function achieved by the operation does not change, or deteriorates very slowly. Paleness of the disc slowly increases. The retina frequently remains attached and no perceptible traction problems in the retinal periphery are to be registered either, because everything has been radically cleared away there. In short, it is obvious that the problems do not come from the posterior segment. If the ciliary body and the space in front of the ora serrata are examined, more or less progressed signs of a flat fibrotic proliferation are to be found, which frequently encloses the entire ciliary body and partly effects the iris. At the early stage the connection to the perforation scar is sometimes still noticeable, later often only a circular fibrotic ring enclosing the whole ciliary body is to be seen. This development in the eyes already severely damaged in the trauma is only partly explained by the fact that many of these eyes may not have been quite so radically operated in the past, that the ciliary body was not completely separated from the scars and not quite cleared from the fibrotic membranes, and that the diaphragm was cut surgically. We think that the proliferative process in these eyes, in spite of radical surgery, progresses further and, as it does not find scaffolding in the anterior segment any more, spreads out flatly on the perforation scars and seizes the ciliary body. The consequence is the irrepressible bulbus atrophy with the slow loss of function. In this situation, in our opinion, presence of silicone at a certain, later stage is disadvantageous.

As described before, under the silicone a 'dead space' is formed, almost without fluid circulation, which is very promoting for the progress of proliferation. It would be very useful in these cases, after stabilization of the posterior segment and scarring of the retina, to remove the silicone from the eyes as early as possible. Unfortunately, in a great number of these eyes this is not possible because of the pre-existing bad function of the ciliary body. Such a severely damaged eye would immediately collapse after the removal of silicone, in spite of the good situation in the posterior segment. The developed extreme hypotony would be followed by an exudative-inflammatory stage and then a proliferative-scarring stage, with the loss of the eye as consequence. For these reasons vitrectomy with silicone injection has in these eyes only a palliative and temporary value, because it only postpones the loss of the eye. In some of these eyes it is possible to prevent this catastrophic development with appropriate and careful surgery and perhaps with removal of silicone. At present, unfortunately, a surgical therapy of the described situation is not possible. Our every attempt by now to disentangle the ciliary body from the ties of fibrotic tissue has failed because of haemorrhage and renewed proliferation.

Except for the last described form of reproliferation all other forms are surgically treatable. In the following paragraph we shall describe clinical manifestations of specific pathoanatomic groups and their surgical treatment.

Operating under silicone

In the choice of surgical technique in all cases of reproliferation the decisive question is whether the operation will be performed under silicone or not. Most manipulations like removal of membranes, retinal surgery or even vitrectomy are easily possible under silicone. Only very extensive vitrectomies with removal of many fibrotic structures are more difficult to perform under silicone. So in the eyes in which the peripheral vitrectomy is not or is only partly performed and in which a longer work with the vitrectome can be expected as well as more haemorrhages, we replace silicone with saline, complete the entire work under saline and subsequently inject silicone. Another reason for us to remove silicone temporarily before the operation is if the patient has been operated somewhere else with for us unfamiliar silicone. Mixing of various sorts of silicone may postoperatively lead to opacifying of silicone, which, although frequently temporary, is optically unpleasant.

In the aphakic eyes the operation begins with inserting of infusion with silicone oil. The use of a little thicker, 1 mm cannula, is convenient because of its larger lumen, but not absolutely necessary. For the operation which is not expected to last too long old sclerotomies may be used. With complicated operations, which take a long time, it is better to make new sclerotomies. Old sclerotomies are namely easily torn further with exchange of instruments, which results in permanent leaking of silicone during the operation. After opening of sclerotomies the flute needle is introduced first and with simultaneous rising of intraocular pressure by injecting of silicone the fluid, which is nearly always to be found in front of the disc, is evacuated. It is important that before one starts any manipulation silicone is in contact with the retina. Another rule for the operation under silicone is that the intraocular pressure is low with each action. The low intraocular pressure allows every manipulation under silicone. With the low intraocular pressure cohesive forces of silicone take care that the silicone bubble with every manipulation on the bottom of the eye, e.g. with pulling on the retina or with removal of membranes, draws back upward leaving space for manipulating. With the high intraocular pressure, on the other hand, no space is left and with manipulating the surface tension is broken and silicone very easily gets under the retina. The intraocular pressure can be regulated with the silicone injection pump, which is connected to the eye by the infusion tube. Injecting of silicone is put in action by the foot pedal of the pump when necessary and also stopped in the same way. The intraocular pressure is not regulated or controlled instrumentally. The only control is the visual control of the surgeon. With the too low pressure the cornea will fold with movements of the bulbus and immediately optically disturb the view. By injecting a little silicone the pressure can be brought to the desired level. The too high pressure is best to be noticed on the blood circulation. The increased pressure with the operation, particularly with the endodrainage is not completely avoidable. When observing pulsation of the blood vessels and certainly with the stop of circulation, injecting of silicone should be interrupted immediately. The best and fastest relief of the too high pressure is taking out of one or both instruments from the eye. Through the open sclerotomies the silicone will flow away and the pressure will be regulated spontaneously.

The optical situation with this operation is mostly optimum. Optical disturbances which sometimes occur are, first, the clouding of the cornea epithelium, then, the prolapsing of silicone through the pupil opening, and finally, too much opacified fluid between the silicone bubble and the retina. Removal of the epithelium will solve the first problem. The astigmatism of the prolapsed silicone is, as already described, best to be solved by suction of the aqueous and bringing of the silicone in a better contact with the cornea. The third problem occurs mostly only at the beginning of the operation and is directly solved with suction of the fluid.

The contact with the retina, and small and slow fluctuation of intraocular pressure as well as excellent visibility are qualities which characterize surgery under silicone as very appropriate for this kind of operations. In the redetachment due to reproliferation a part of the retina is often still attached at the reoperation and needs no surgery. While the surgery under water, due to water turbulence and frequent fluctuation of the pressure combined with manipulating on the detached retina, may cause detachment of the attached retina, with the surgery under silicone this is practically impossible. Silicone fixes, so to say, the given situation and with skilled manipulating makes the whole operation easier.

Regarding the described basic principles for surgery under silicone, the following step of the operation is examining and assessing the situation in the eye. In idiopathic retinal detachments with PVR and giant tears the pathoanatomical pictures of a redetachment after reproliferation hardly differ and can be described together.

As the periphery in correctly operated eyes as a rule offers no problems, attention is concentrated on the centre, where usually three kinds of changes dominate the picture. First, the epiretinal membranes, which often, particularly with the giant tears, are concentrated in the macula area, further, shortening of the retina due to forming of fibrotic membranes at the edge of the circular buckle, and as last, subretinal proliferations. The operative course and the elimination of causes of the detachment should follow in this order. As the mobility and shortening of the retina can only be assessed after removal of epiretinal membranes, the given order is logical and can be used in most cases. Epiretinal membranes can relatively easily be removed with the short spatula and later with the forceps. When they are situated more peripherally, they mostly spread as far as the edges of the buckle, where they pass into vast scars and are difficult to remove. Also at this stage they should be removed only so far, because the retina would tear at the edge at a further attempt. One tries first to clean the entire retina centrally. In areas where the retina is not covered with mature membranes, the pigment sediment and yet immature membranes are not seldom found. This part of the retina has also to be cleaned, best with the scratcher and the flute needle. In these cases the detachment is mostly flat and the retina is not folded, which makes the cleaning considerably easier. Nevertheless, little haemorrhages are very frequent, particularly at the edges of scars, because the vulnerability of the retina is increased in second operations. The blood has to be sucked out immediately and the bleeding sites coagulated. After cleaning of the retina the mobility can be assessed. With the drainage of subretinal fluid it will be shown immediately whether the retina tends to attach. One tries to use the old holes for endodrainage; if there are none, the retina is opened at the edge of the buckle. Generally even before the drainage it is to be seen whether the retina is shortened or not. Those retinas that are elevated most at the edge of the buckle after removal of epiretinal membranes, are also shortened by traction and will not attach after the endodrainage. However, it is worth trying. Some retinas can be attached or nearly attached by increasing of the intraocular pressure and by endodrainage. Yet this has little use because it is not the real situation and the attachment is achieved only with the pressure of silicone. When later the pressure decreases, the retina will be detached again. Therefore the mobility of the retina should be definitely assessed under the low pressure and after the drainage. A retina not attached in this way will remain detached and cannot be left so. There are two therapeutic possibilities to solve this situation. The first is to try to remove the fibrotic membranes and structures with the scars on the buckle, which very rarely succeeds. The fibrotic structures are very adherent to the scars and are very difficult to remove. In this attempt the retina will mostly tear and haemorrhages are also unavoidable. The second possibility is a retinotomy by which the clean retina is separated from the buckle and proliferative structures. In most cases this is by far the best solution. The retina is first diathermized at the end of the buckle and separated from the periphery with a blunt

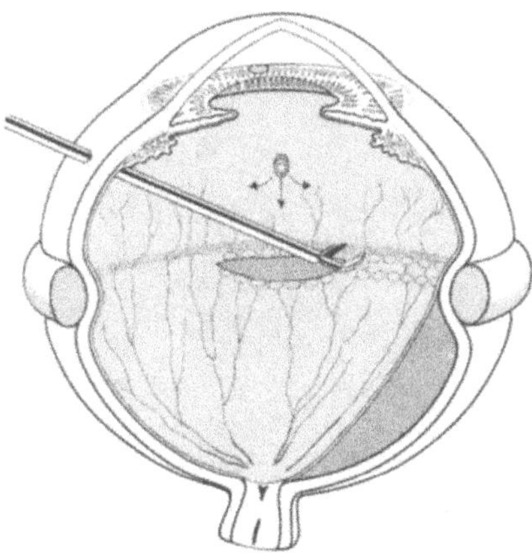

Figure 1. Relaxing retinotomy after diathermocoagulation under silicone oil.

instrument at the site of diathermy. A long row of diathermic coagulates can be done at once and then the separation of the retina with the vitrectome or motorized scissors performed (Fig. 1). It is less important which instrument is used than to attempt to avoid bleeding. After the separation of one part of the retina, the necrotized retina, blood and subretinal fluid should be removed with the flute needle immediately. At the same time it is also an additional test whether the retina is relieved and tends to attach. The retinotomy had better be large than small, in any case it should reach as far as the attached retina. The best sign that the retinotomy is long enough is the complete attachment of the retina. The space created between the central edge of the retina and the buckle, which is the larger the more the retina is shortened, should be cleaned from the debris and blood rests. If necessary the edges of the retina should be coagulated again to prevent later bleeding. This holds in particular in case that cryopexy has been used. Finally, the edges of the retinotomy should be coagulated, best with the endolaser. If after the removal of epiretinal membranes it is obvious that subretinal proliferations are the cause of the detachment as well, they should also be removed. With isolated strands and with a retina that is not shortened, this should be done through a small central retinotomy. Yet this is seldom the case, because the subretinal proliferation is mostly the sign of a long existing detachment and frequently combined with the above-mentioned shortening of the retina. In this case the removal should be combined with a large relaxing retinotomy. The retinotomy should be done in the same way as described above. After finishing the retinotomy and coagulation of the edges the retina should be rolled up like a carpet from the periphery to the centre. This is done best with the brush needle, with which the retina is sucked up easily. The intraocular pressure should be a little increased (with a correctly performed retinotomy, when the retina is not under traction

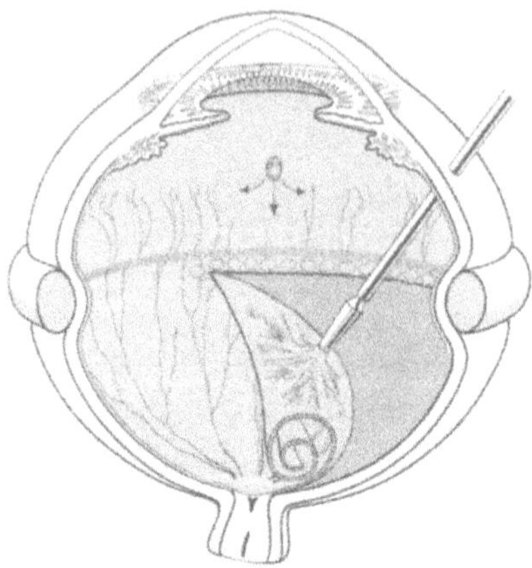

Figure 2. Removal of subretinal proliferations after the retinotomy and rolling up of the retina under silicone oil.

any more, one need not fear that the silicone will get under the retina with the slightly increased pressure). The retina rolled up in this way will gradually not only enable free view on the subretinal space but also on the retinal back surface (Fig. 2). The removal of the subretinal structures and cleaning of the subretinal space does not present any difficulty. When this has been done, unrolling of the retina should follow in the opposite direction. This should also be done gradually and carefully without pulling immediately at the end of the retina. If this manipulation is not done step by step and slowly, the silicone can get behind the retina more easily. The best instrument is the blunt membrane peeler, with which the retina cannot be damaged easily. When the retina has been reposed, the edges should be further treated in the above described way.

In the detachments with PVR after perforating injuries we find, although often localized differently, roughly the same pathoanatomical changes as with the two first described groups. An additional and characteristic change is the reproliferation from the perforation scars. Also the other changes like epiretinal membranes and particularly subretinal proliferations often have their origin in the perforation scars. This fact obliges to pay the greatest attention to the proliferation scar during the operation. After the removal of epiretinal membranes the retina will frequently appear to be shortened or folded by the traction coming from the scar. Therefore a retinotomy should be made around the scar and in this way the scar separated from the retina. As it has already been described with traumatic detachments, it is very important to create a large space between the central edge of the retina and the scar so as to avoid a possible traction in future. Subsequently, if subretinal strands exist, which very often come from the scar, they can be removed by retinotomy. If the performed circumcision of the scar is too small for it, the retinotomy should be

150

extended in the desired direction. The further treatment does not differ from
the above described one.

The reproliferation in the diabetic traction detachment shows, in its clinical
manifestation, many differences from the three first described groups. As
neither the same primary disease nor the same proliferative process are
concerned, this picture is a combination of the original disease and the PVR.
So as with the first operation, new developed changes after the reproliferation
are concentrated in the centre and sometimes come from the disc. Basically,
there are two kinds of proliferative membranes. The first are the delicate
transparent membranes, with which the starting point is difficult to locate and
which cover the entire fundus. Further characteristics are the enormous
spreading – practically the entire fundus is covered with them – and the
relatively low inclination to contraction through which the retina is not much
folded either. It concerns completely new membranes, developed often surprisingly short after the first operation, which is proved by the fact that under
the membranes one can frequently discover old diathermy coagulates (particularly in new cases). The membranes are elastic, do not break easily and
because they are not fast attached to the retina, are relatively easy to remove.
The other kind are the whitish fibrotic membranes, sometimes vascularized,
which very often start from the old scars or retinotomies and are very strong.
The mixture of both kinds is not frequent. The third, fortunately rare form is
the explosion-like reproliferation in young diabetics often preceded by postoperative haemorrhages where the old blood has not been removed in time.
The starting point is mostly the site of the blood clot, but the reproliferation
spreads out behind the silicone bubble on the whole retina and sometimes the
periphery is affected as well.

In the first form there is often a total flat detachment without many folds and
after the removal of membranes the retina is often attached without surgical
measures. The second form often causes only a local detachment and looks
rather harmless before the operation. Yet during the operation one frequently
discovers that one cannot manage without retinal surgery, retinotomy and
sometimes also retinectomy. Subsequently, the retina is mostly attached easily
under the silicone. In the third form an extensive retinal surgery is mostly
necessary to free the retina from the fibrotic membranes. Yet in these eyes the
final success is very rare, and due to continuous reproliferations the eye
perishes after all. It is especially important to remember that in this group
prevention of bleeding and cleaning of the fundus of the eye at the end of the
operation have a very particular significance for the prevention of reproliferation.

All these forms of reproliferation in the various groups that we have
discussed by now concern the eyes operated in the usual way after the
described surgical principles. Lately, as the use of silicone has increased

enormously, we see more and more cases in which silicone was injected after very incomplete vitrectomy combined with the retinal surgery. In these cases the retina was not cleaned and the fibrotic structures were not at all or only incompletely removed. To achieve attachment of the retina at the end of the operation the retinal surgery was often applied and the retina often fixed with tacks. In such cases the reproliferation starts immediately after the operation, because the membranes and other fibrotic structures have not been removed. The scars of the retinopexy have no time at all to develop and to fix the retina, because due to the proliferative process the traction can take its course immediately after the operation and detach the retina, which was mechanically fixed in the operation. Due to the presence of silicone in the eye there is no place for the retina to detach freely, on the other hand the proliferative membranes, by their contraction, pull the retina which has been cut surgically and tear it further behind the silicone. In this way bizarre clinical pictures develop, which we never saw before the application of silicone. Huge holes develop with silicone behind the contracted retina, or the retina is to be seen in front of the disc, entirely shrunken like a lump. These cases are mostly inoperable and as such warn against the lay use of silicone oil and retinal surgery.

In the end the question of the right time for reoperation should be discussed. As we have seen, the first group, the idiopathic detachment with PVR and the giant tears have approximately the same postoperative course. The patho-anatomical changes that have caused redetachment develop relatively slowly and the detachment slowly increases. This is a favourable development for planning of an operation, which allows us, with the regular follow-up of the patient, to choose the right time for the operation. As it is never certain that the following operation will be the last, and that one will succeed to stop the process by the operation, it is better to postpone the surgery as long as possible. In this way a certain maturing of the proliferative membranes will occur, which then become better visible and easier to remove, which again increases chances for the final success. The waiting, though, should not be done at the expense of the function and therefore the patient should be followed up in short intervals. If the macula is attached and the process takes place in the inferior periphery, it should be tried to postpone the operation for 4–6 weeks.

It is entirely different with the diabetic traction detachment. There the development is frequently much faster and less predictable. Besides, the proliferation is much more often localized in the very centre and the function is frequently endangered already in the beginning. For all these reasons these patients should be operated as soon as possible.

Evacuation of the silicone

Even before one starts discussing the problem of evacuation of the silicone the question should be put whether and why the silicone should be removed from the eye. In our patient population we have quite a few successfully operated patients who have had silicone in the eye for 7–8 years and even one patient from the first period who has had silicone in the eye for nearly 20 years. In all these patients the function of the eye has remained more or less the same and no complications have appeared. All these patients are aphakic and not vitrectomized, and the silicone is incapsulated with the vitreous and fibrotic membranes and so completely separated from the anterior segment. Many have a stationary peripheral detachment, but the central retina is attached and functioning. In practically all of them the other eye is good and they see no reason to be operated on further. There is even a considerable number of patients in whom the operation failed at that time. Many have a mature cataract and still, as immediately after the operation, the positive light perception. These eyes are not irritated, as a rule, and cause the patients no trouble. Clinically, the silicone, at least that one we have used, seems to have no toxical effect on the eye. The problems begin when silicone gets in the anterior segment and when it begins emulsifying. As in course of years we have so changed the surgical technique for the reasons mentioned here several times, that the emulsification of silicone is almost unavoidable, it is advisable, if possible, to remove silicone from the eye. Beside the reason to remove silicone so as to prevent complications, there is another practical-logistic point of view to do so. Namely, as long as the patient has silicone in the eye, he is a patient and should be followed-up regularly. After the successful evacuation of silicone and a reasonable follow-up period, this obligation ceases for both the patient and the surgeon. The difficulty is that the evacuation of silicone always involves the risk of redetachment, which makes choice of time for this operation extremely difficult. As everybody knows there are no dependable parameters which could show when the proliferative process has burnt out and stopped. This situation will possibly never be reached in the eye and a latent danger to wake up the process again is probably always present. The first condition for the removal of silicone is the complete attachment of the retina for a longer time. A precise time is difficult to indicate and from experience it depends very much on the etiology of the case, course of disease, number of operations and appearance of the fundus. The minimum time after which silicone can be removed from the eye would be, with exceptions, roughly about 3 weeks. In the most favourable position are the diabetic eyes, which due to very small inclination to reproliferations may not need silicone, in a favourable case, already after a few weeks. The other extreme are the eyes after perforating injuries, especially with hypotony and damages in the anterior segment, which in spite of long complete attachment of the retina develop a phthisis bulbi after removal of silicone. It is obvious from the above-described that a selection with pre-examination should take place before evacuation of silicone. It is another question whether a preparation of the eye in the sense of a photocoagulation should be done before the evacuation. As the relative security achieved in this way has always to be paid with a part of the function, we have not yet applied photocoagulation as a routine procedure with all patients. We have neither done a statistic evaluation between coagulated and not coagulated eyes and therefore can only say to have the impression that the laser light coagulation performed before evacuation of silicone decreases the risk of redetachment.

Silicone can be removed from the eye in different ways. The simplest way is to connect the eye with the infusion and to wash out the silicone from the eye through a corneal opening or through a sclerotomy. Yet we prefer a controlled evacuation with the active suction of the silicone. The advantages are a perfect control of the intraocular pressure, an optically controlled evacuation of the main bubble and subsequently also optically controlled washing out of small emulsified bubbles from the eye. An additional advantage in this method is the possibility to perform vitrectomy immediately afterwards, which is very useful in the not vitrectomized eyes.

For evacuation of silicone we use the silicone vacuum pump. After inserting of infusion a sclerotomy is done. For suction we mostly use a 1.2 mm thick cannula with the opening on the side. As the pump has a strong suction power it is very important that the cannula is always well connected to the silicone bubble for which the side opening of the cannula is advantageous. One starts with suction only when one has ensured that the cannula is inserted in the middle of the silicone bubble. It is very important to pay attention that the cannula is in good contact with silicone during the whole procedure. With suction the bubble will become smaller and raise from the bottom of the eye. The size of the bubble and the distance to the posterior pole can be tested by pressing the edge of the bubble from inside with the tip of the cannula. Deformation of the silicone bubble developed in this way will manifest itself on the change of the interfacial reflex. Finally the silicone bubble will become wholly visible in the pupilar opening hanging on the suction cannula until it completely disappears. After removal of the main silicone bubble many small bubbles frequently remain in the eye. These can be removed with the appropriate suction power of the vitrectome. It is practically impossible to remove all small bubbles from the eye, particularly because many have settled behind the iris and in the vitreous and membrane remnants. Therefore it is advantageous to have the possibility of vitrectomy at hand to remove them further. With the examination of the eye fundus it will sometimes be found out that the retina is covered with bubbles. If one tries to suck the bubbles out with the

154

flute needle, one will sometimes find that the entire retina is covered with an extremely fine membrane stretched directly in front of the retina like a cobweb. The small silicone bubbles are between the membrane and the retina and after removal of the membrane they are easy to wash away from the retinal surface. The membranes tear very easily and at removal they are only grown fast at the edge of the buckle. The development of these membranes is not clear to us. As they are often pigmented it is possible that old epiretinal membranes are concerned, which are not active any more and have lost their contractibility. The small silicone bubbles could then get between the membranes and the retina through holes in the membranes which are sometimes visible. Anyhow, we cannot remember a redetachment to which we could ascribe the activity of these membranes. Another discovery is sometimes the epiretinal membranes which are completely white and can be peeled away from the retina without difficulty. The whole procedure of evacuation of the silicone takes 15–20 min and in most eyes this time is sufficient to remove the greatest part of the emulsified bubbles. In the eyes with the normal intraocular pressure the rest of the bubbles will disappear spontaneously after some time.

Plate 8. Postoperative course. Complications after silicone tamponade.

1. Silicone keratopathy.
2. Mature cataract and a freely floating silicone bubble in the anterior chamber (AC).
3. Beginning subcapsular cataract after vitrectomy and silicone tamponade.
4. Freely floating silicone bubble in the AC after vitrectomy and silicone tamponade. Giant tear with pseudophaky.
5. Emulsified silicone in the AC with the vertical position of the head.
6. Emulsified silicone in the chamber angle.

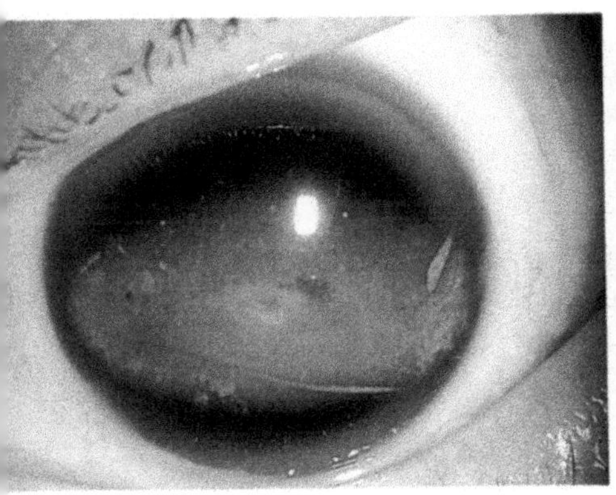
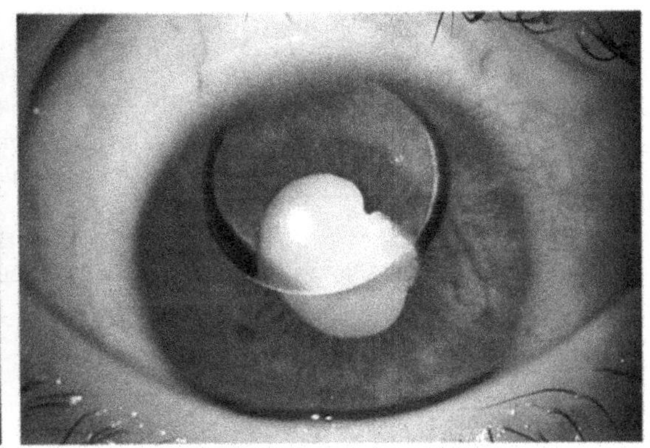

2

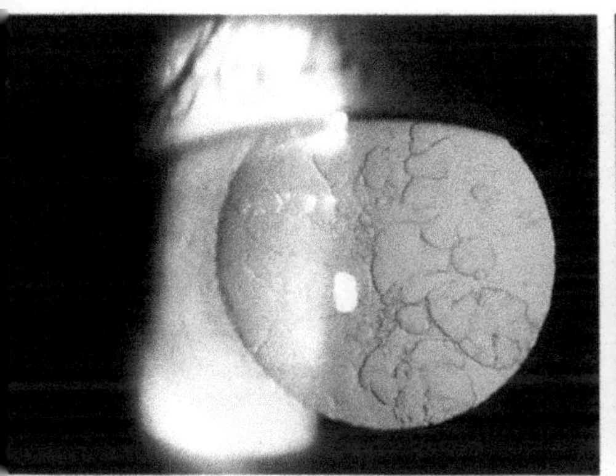
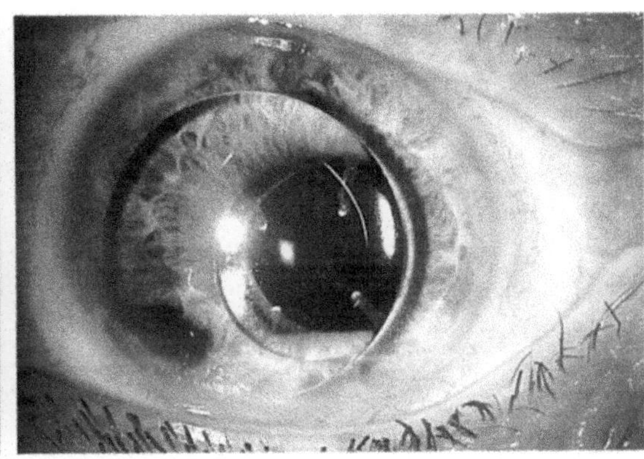

4

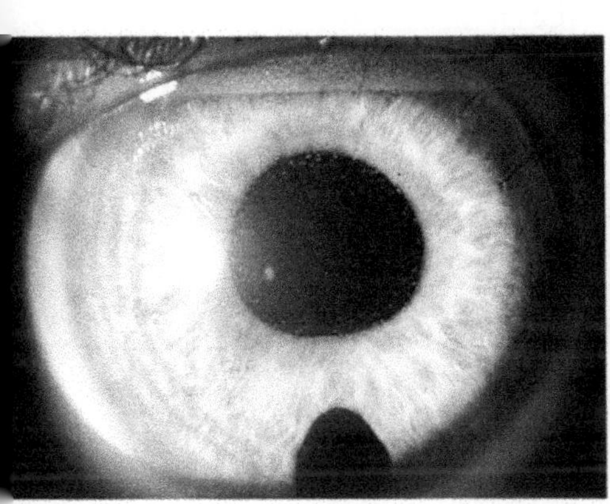
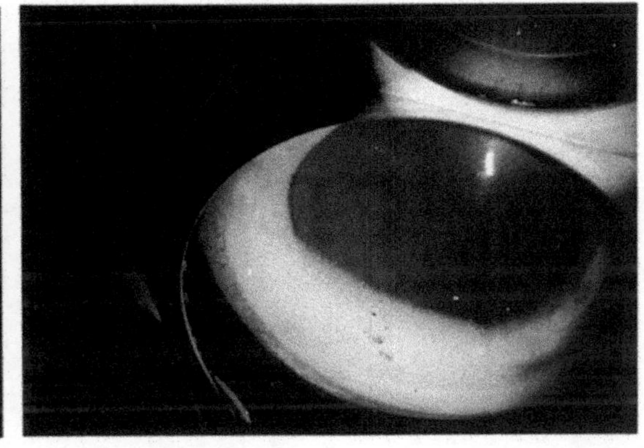

6

Plate 9. Postoperative course. Miscellaneous.

1. A small silicone bubble separated from the main bubble by residual membranes.
2. Emulsified silicone between the main bubble and the retina.
3. Emulsified silicone behind the retina. Paramacular hole.
4. Functioning 6 o'clock iridectomy after cataract extraction, vitrectomy and silicone tamponade.
5. Surgical widening of the pupil in pseudophaky. Silicone tamponade, 6 o'clock iridectomy.
6. A small silicone bubble remained after removal of silicone.

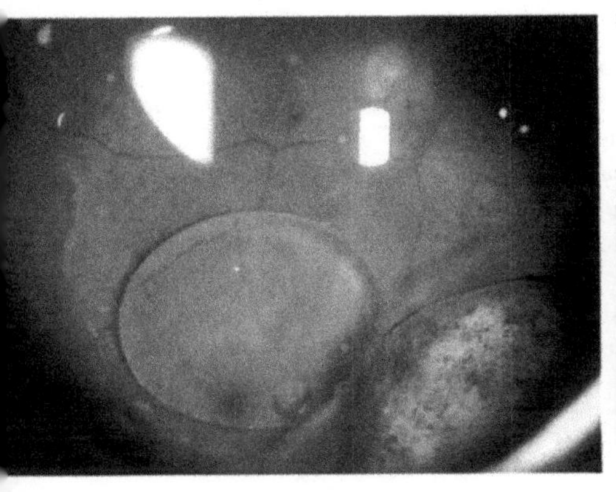
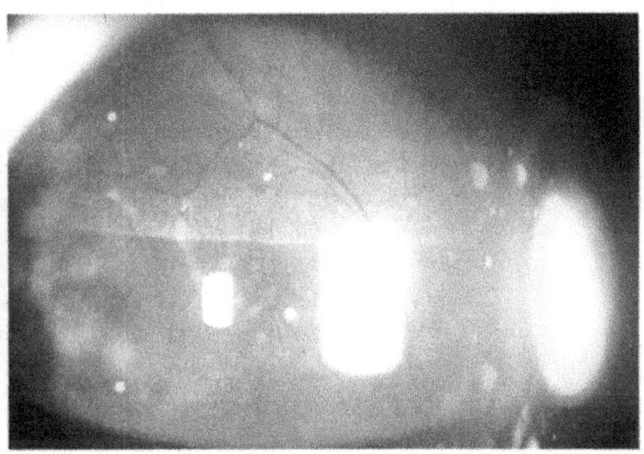

2

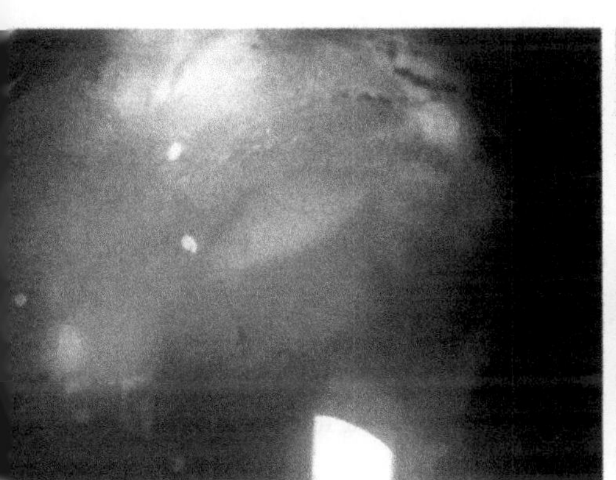
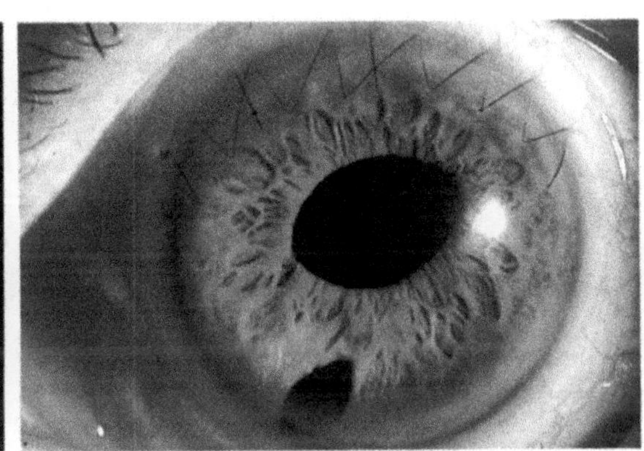

4

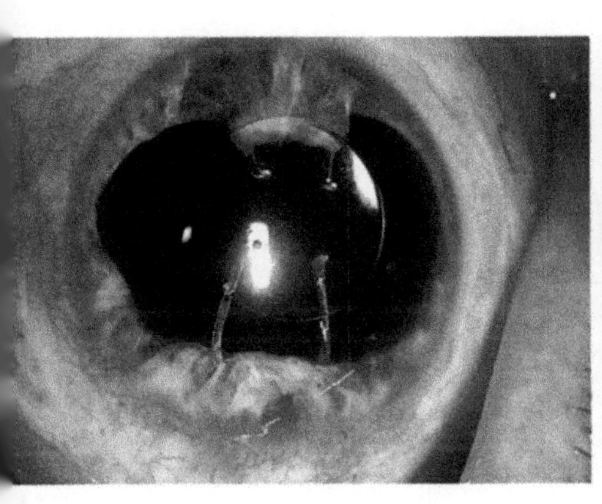
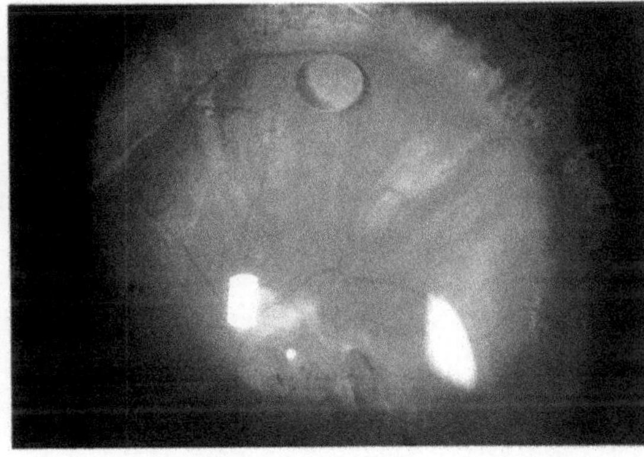

6

Plate 10. Postoperative course. Persisting of PVR.

1. Traction detachment with PVR after a dubble perforating injury.
2. Situation after the successful operation: vitrectomy, circumcision of the perforation scar, silicone tamponade. VOD: 0,1 (see visual field).
3. Situation after the second operation. Repeated reproliferation. Epiretinal membranes with traction on the retina. No detachment. Visual field strongly deteriorated (see visual field).
4. Two years after the first operation. In spite of a third operation reproliferation cannot be stopped. Pale disc.
5. Four years after the first operation. Final situation is reached. Strong scarring, optic nerve atrophy, the partly avascular retina. The retina detached. Visual field strongly deteriorated.
6. Idem.

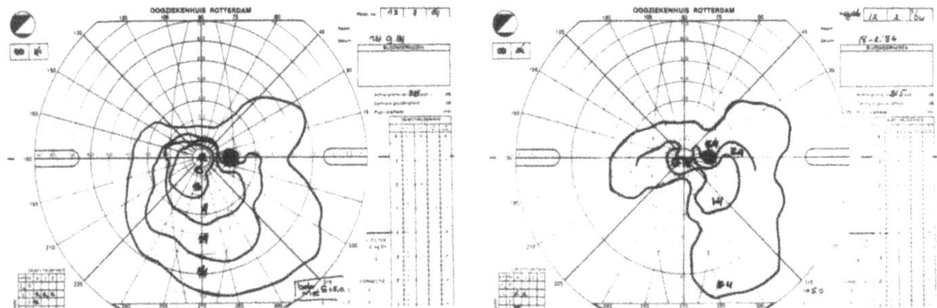

Visual field belonging to plate 10.2.　　　Visual field belonging to plate 10.3.

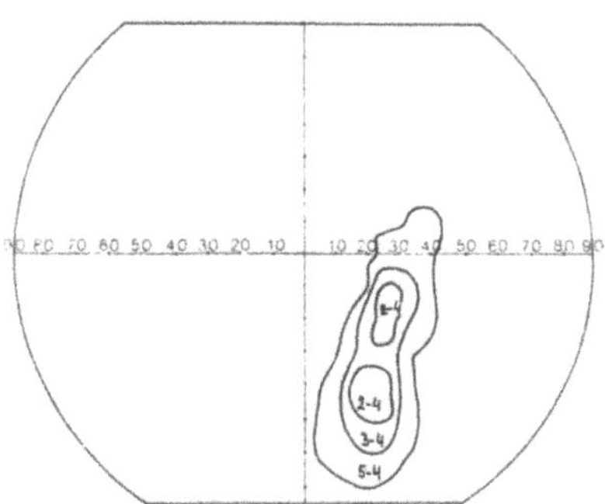

Visual field belonging to plate 10.5.

160

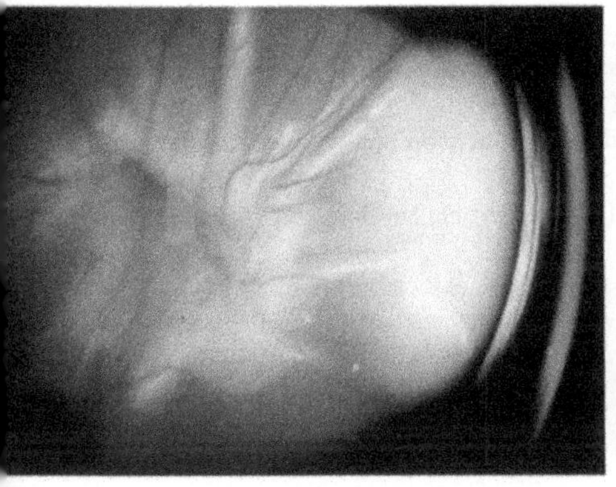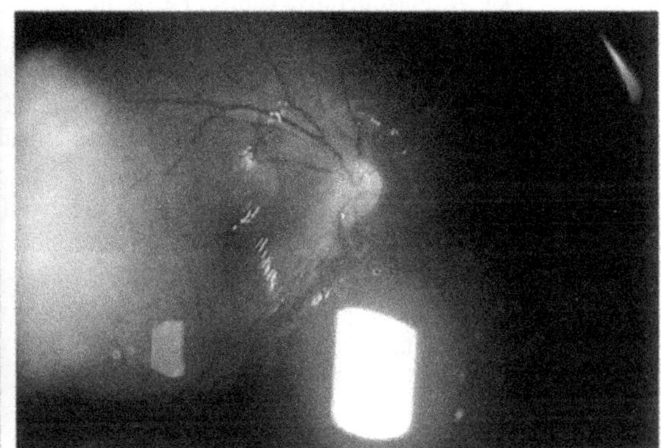

2

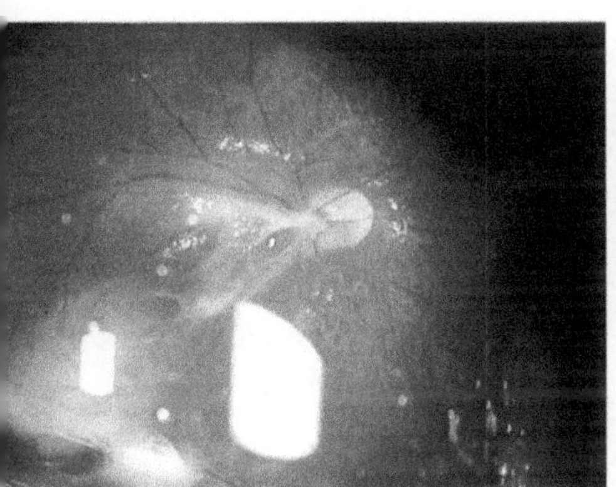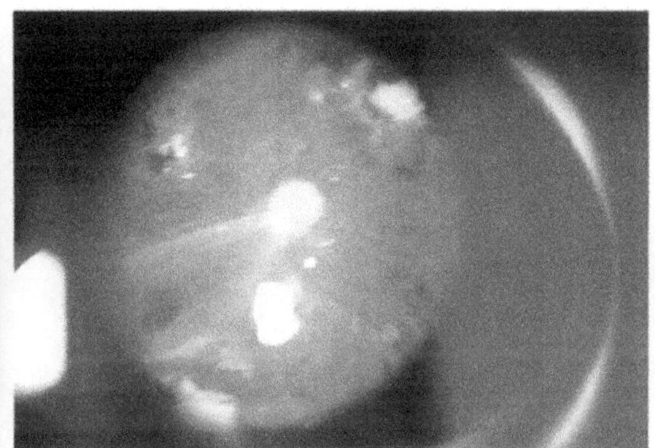

4

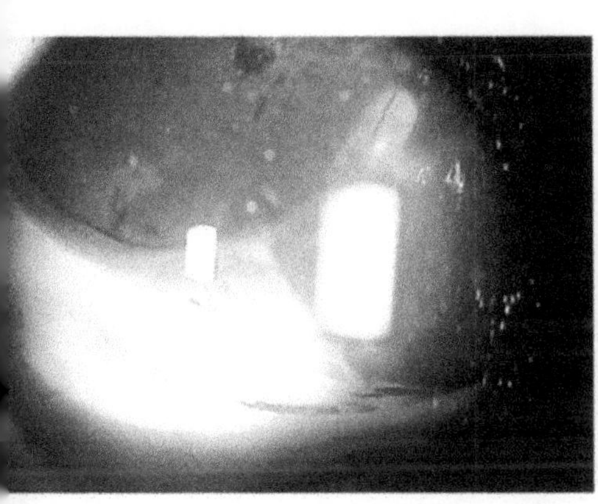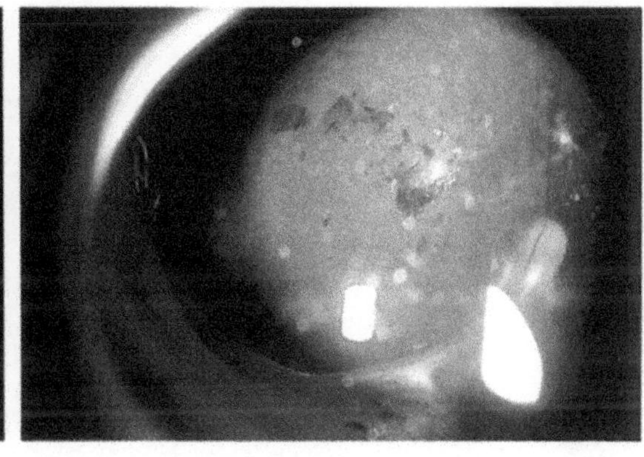

6

Plate 11. Postoperative course. Persisting of PVR.

1. Situation after vitrectomy, cataract extraction and silicone tamponade. Reproliferation a week after the operation. Massive subretinal proliferation.
2. Situation after reoperation – retinotomy and removal of subretinal proliferation under silicone.
3. Reproliferation a few weeks after successful vitrectomy and silicone tamponade. Epi- and subretinal proliferation in the posterior pole.
4. Situation after reoperation – removal of epi- and subretinal membranes.
5. A slowly progressing subretinal proliferation with subsequent detachment in the inferior part, 6 months after the operation.
6. Reproliferation in inferior part of the retina. Opening of an old tear due to traction.

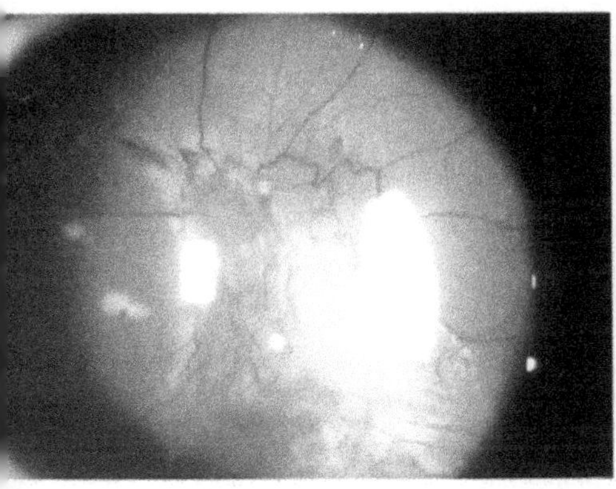
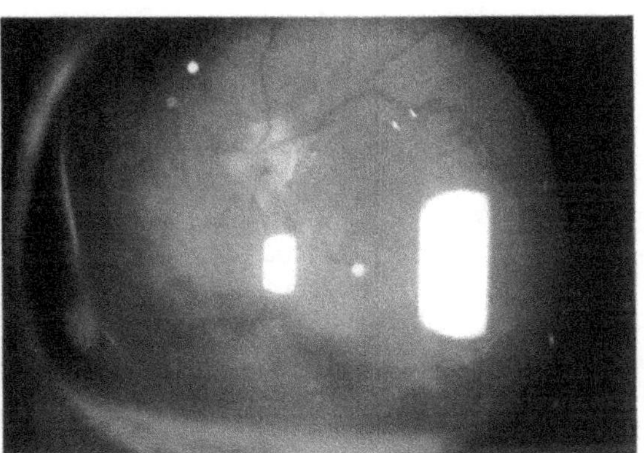

2

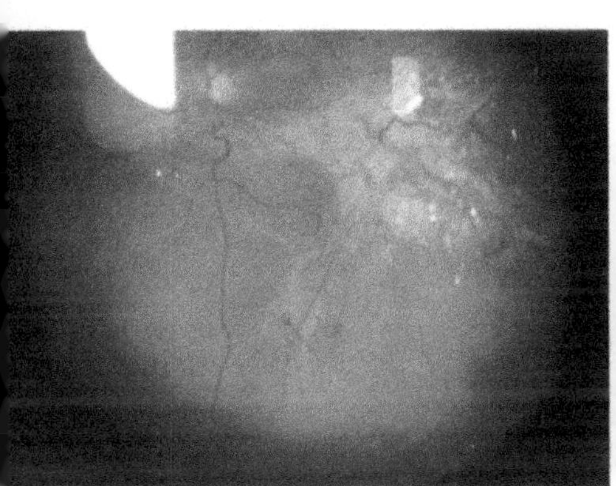
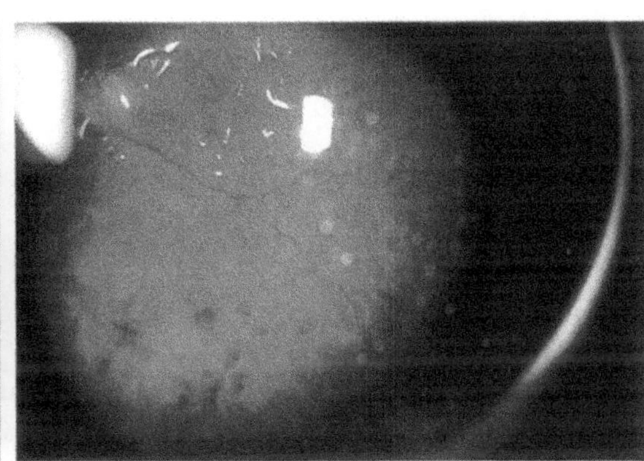

4

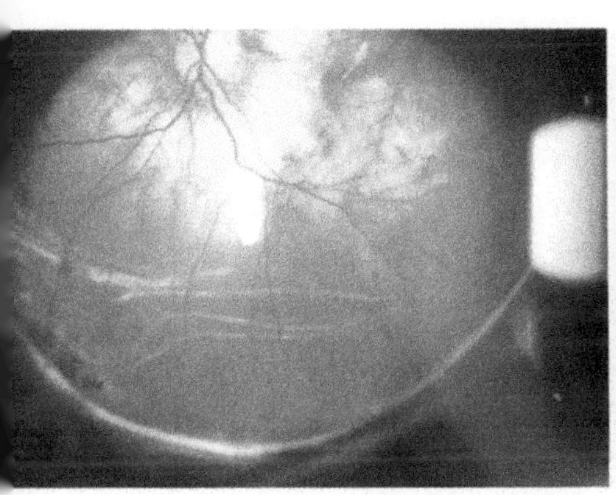
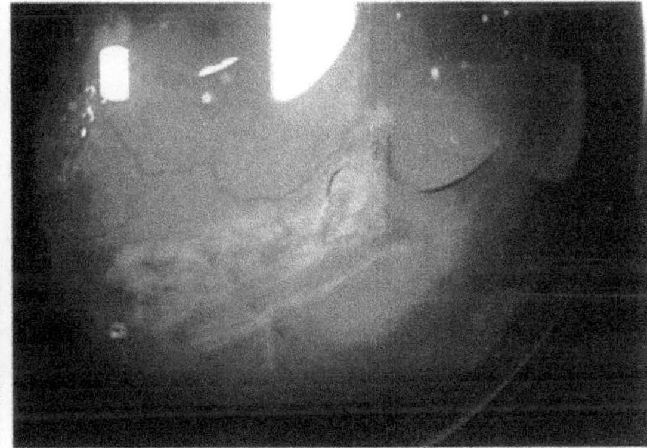

6

Plate 12. Postoperative course. Persisting of PVR. Complications of retinal surgery.

  1. Situation after a severe perforating injury with traumatic aniridy, aphaky and total detachment.

  2. Vitrectomy and silicone tamponade. Except for local residual epiretinal membranes the retina is attached.

3+4. The same case. Reproliferation and fibrotic organisation of the ciliary body. The retina is completely attached. No activity in the posterior segment. Slow phthisis bulbi with very slow deterioration of the function in spite of the silicone tamponade.

  5. Enlarging of the iatrogenic hole due to reproliferation following an incomplete vitrectomy and membrane peeling. The consequence of inadequate use of retinal surgery and silicone tamponade.

  6. Total shrinking of the retina in front of the disc after retinotomy and silicone tamponade. The consequence of use of retinal surgery in the contracted and unclean retina.

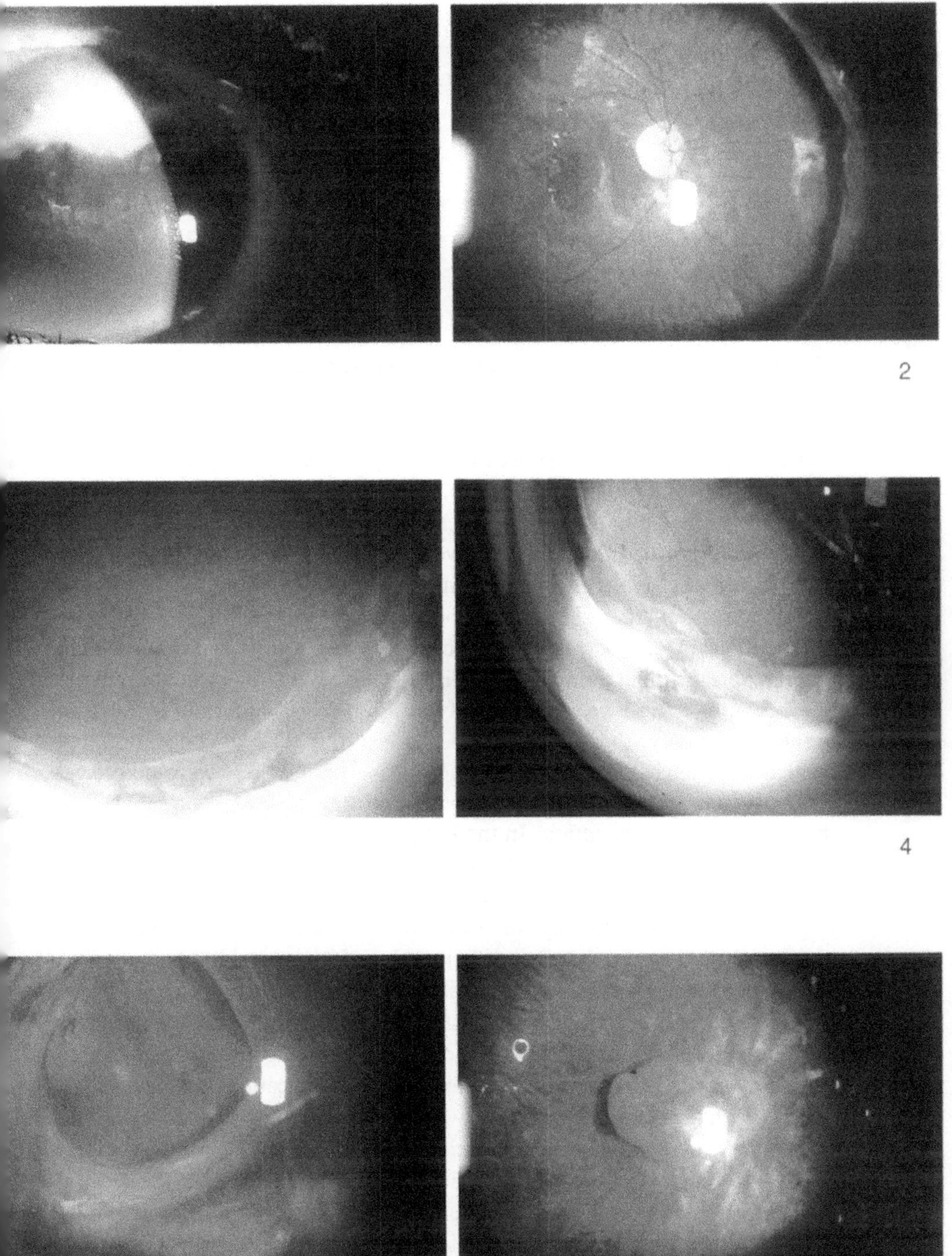

2

4

165 6

9. Results

The statistic compilation of the results in this surgery is even more difficult than otherwise, and while an abundance of facts is revealed, many remain hidden.

In this pathology, in which the cases are very difficult to compare, the course of disease and the prognosis of single cases depend on so many factors, the decision, the manipulation and the technical means of the surgeons play such an important part for the postoperative course and final result, all particular statistics are of a relative value and only conditionally usable.

However, the statistical evaluation of the results is an unavoidable necessity for the clinical work, and therefore we want to give a survey of the results in several tables without going into details too much. With the evaluation of the first 6 months of 1985 we want to satisfy various aspects important for such an evaluation. Firstly, that is the period in which our surgical conception had been applied unchanged for some time. In that period there were no radical technical changes and all operations were performed by three surgeons after the same surgical conception. In the last years the number of operations has stabilized on the level in the tables, which has allowed us to evaluate a sufficient number of about 250 consecutive operations from a relatively short interval of 6 months. Finally, the evaluated period gives us also the opportunity of the follow-up of more than 18 months, which is considerably sufficient time to get the impression about stability of the results.

As we are of the opinion that all statistics on the results in the posterior segment surgery are very deficient and much concealing if they do not quote the number of patients with the same surgical indications who were not operated on in the same interval, we have registered these as well. The surprisingly small number of four patients excluded from the primary operation perhaps needs to be explained. As we have written in detail on the surgical indications before, we only want to add that we regarded the positive light perception as the minimum condition for an indication for surgery. Existing or not existing of a correct light projection was found more or less important in connection with other clinical findings, and if not existing mostly not found negative as such and seldom an excluding indication for surgery. After these very widely interpreted indications for surgery only four patients were excluded from surgery although they would come into consideration for the operation after the usual criterium. This occurred because the patients refrained from the operation after the interview or the operation was not advisable for reason of their health. This small number can be explained for the greatest part with the fact that our own patient population has traditionally a positive and confident attitude towards the treatment and very rarely refrain from the further treatment themselves. With the patients referred to us a selected group is concerned, for whom, for various reasons, indications for surgery leave little choice (e.g. monophthalmia).

The other group in Table 3 are the cases which during the primary operation were found inoperable and abandoned as such. In the last few years, because of the strongly increased number of operations, we have decided not to operate any more the cases in which, in our experience, very bad functional prognosis is combined with several operations. Such cases are mostly to be found in the group of detachments following severe perforating traumas. The

Table 1. Operations 1-1-1985–1-1-1986 (N = 1157).

Conventional surgery (buckling)	457
Vitrectomy	178
Silicone surgery	522
Total	1157

Table 2. Consecutive silicone operations 1-1-1985–1-7-1985 (N = 257).

Primary silicone operation	134
Refill	84
Silicone removal	39
Total	257

Table 3.

Excluded from primary surgery	4
Abandoned at primary operation	9
(incalculated in detached cases in Table 5)	

other eye in these patients is mostly normal and undamaged, which makes the decision much easier not to operate the concerned eye any more. As it is not possible to decide before the operation, in particular with the traumatized eyes, whether an operation is sensible or not, this decision is made during the operation after a preliminary interview with the patient. Nine patients in the table belong to such cases and are incalculated in failures in further tables.

Further our interest goes to the primary operated patients (Table 2) and to the cases in which silicone was removed. The reoperated patients in whom silicone was refilled are more difficult to evaluate and they only illustrate the high number of reoperations of 30–40% in the total statistics. In the primary operated cases the distribution on various indication groups was representative for the daily clinical work (Table 4). The results given in Table 5 are the final results after the follow-up of approximately 6 months, but before removal of silicone. The cases with residual detachments (5 – Table 5) are operated in the further course of the follow-up and presented in Table 7. In Table 7 it is conspicuous that the complete attachment of the retina has been achieved in a great percentage of the patients (40–50%) only after two or more operations. At the same time it can also be said that the eyes once operated successfully or partly successfully, even if the half only after several operations, have preserved the anatomical success. The functional results in Table 6 are the final results after the follow-up of 18 months. The functional results immediately following the first operation are not evaluated, but we know they were much

Table 4. Primary silicone surgery (vitrectomy + silicone injection) (N = 134).

PVR after idiop. detach.	66
Giant tears	16
Traum. detach.	16
Diabet. traction detach.	36
Total	134

Table 5. Results of primary silicone surgery (vitrectomy + silicone injection) (N = 134).

	Attached	Partly att.	Detached	Unknown	Total
PVR – idiop. detach.	53	5	6	2	66
Giant tears	14	–	1	1	16
Traum. detach.	13	–	3	–	16
Diabet. trac. detach.	28	–	7	1	36
Total	108 ±80%	5 ±4%	17 ±13%	4 ±3%	134 ±100%

better and deteriorated at average in 18 months. It is certain that the anatomical success after several operations has to be paid by significant loss of function. This is also proved by a great number of cases without light perception after the operation (13) in Table 6. On the other hand it is very encouraging to see that about one third (46) successfully operated patients still has reached visual acuity of 0.1–0.15. Satisfactorily small is also the number of patients lost for the follow-up (4) (Tables 5 and 6) in spite of many referred patients coming from abroad.

Summing up one could say that certainly the anatomical results but also the functional ones are satisfactory. It must be mentioned at the same time that in the high percentage of the successfully operated patients those are concerned

Table 6. V.A. after primary silicone surgery (N = 134).

	No L.P.	L.P.–H.M.	C.F.	0.1–0.15	>0.15	Un-known	Total
PVR – idiop. detach.	5	14	19	26	1	1	66
Giant tears	1	3	6	6	–	–	16
Traum. detach.	2	3	9	2	–	–	16
Diabet. trac. detach.	5	5	12	8	3	3	36
Total	13	25	46	42	4	4	134

Table 7. Results after primary silicone surgery in 108 attached and 5 partly attached cases after follow-up of more than 18 months (N = 113).

Remained attached after one operation	59
Remained attached after two or more operations	54
Total	113

Table 8. Silicone oil removal (N = 39).

PVR – idiop. detach.	27
Giant tears	5
Trauma	2
Diabetes	5
Total	39

that still have silicone in the eyes and that in some of them it is not yet the final success. The great number of reoperations shows that this success has been paid for with much trouble and sacrifice for the patient but also for the surgeon. It is also to be understood from the great number of patients without light perception after the operation that this complicated and aggressive surgery can ruin the entire function of the eye in case of failure.

The results after evacuation of silicone are a little disappointing. A relatively great number of redetachments of 30–40% (Table 9) has motivated us lately to intensify the preparatory measures (laser coagulation), by which these results have significantly improved in the last time. Nevertheless the risk of redetachment in this final operation cannot be neglected. The redetachment occurs mostly in the period of the intensive postoperative follow-up and the patients can soon be reoperated successfully (Table 11). Yet this disappointing result of the operation expected to be the last is the reason for many patients to refuse further surgery. This is expressed clearly in Table 10.

Table 9. Results after silicone oil removal (N = 39).

Retina attached	23
Retina redetached	16
Total	39

Table 10. Refill after redetachment at silicone oil removal (N = 16).

Retina attached	12
Non operated	4
Total	16

Table 11. V.A. after silicone oil removal and refill after redetachment (N = 35).

	H.M.	C.F.	0.1–0.15	>0.15	Total
Retina attached after removal	2	3	16	2	23
Retina attached after refill	1	7	3	1	12
Total					35

Conclusion

At the end of this book it seems useful to say a few words summing up possibilities, limits and prospects for development of vitreoretinal surgery with silicone tamponade.

It is plausible that the combination of vitrectomy with silicone injection has created a basis for development of retinal surgery. The combination of the three techniques enables us today to treat a considerable number of previously inoperable cases successfully. The best results are achieved when this technique is used at the right moment, i.e. not only after many operations with less promising techniques. The use of this technique is not a universal remedy and favourable and final results have often been achieved only after several operations. Application of this technique, therefore, demands from the surgeon not only clinical insight and usual manual skilfulness but even more perseverance to continue the treatment in spite of, largely, not so encouraging results, and a very close and good relationship with the patients, who are frequently in a pitiful position. The surgeons who use silicone injection only as the last resort, in a single attempt to help the patient (and sometimes themselves) in the desperate situation after a previously failed operation, act in the wrong way. In the long run they will have very bad results and no satisfaction, and finally they will abandon the use of this technique. Bad results achieved in this way cannot, in any case, be attributed to the technique itself.

A relatively small number of patients eligible for this surgery and, on the other hand, a great variety of cases within this number make learning of this technique and building up of clinical experience difficult. For these and for other above-mentioned reasons it seems recommendable to reserve the use of this technique for the centres that have a sufficient number of patients and favourable operating facilities and where several surgeons working together can dedicate themselves to a continuous work with patients.

The improved results achieved through the use of vitrectomy combined with retinal surgery and silicone tamponade, have lately much stimulated spreading of this technique. At the same time, these results have clearly shown therapeutic limits of the technique. As it has been mentioned repeatedly in this book, use of a surgical technique in treatment of consequences of a proliferative process is largely inadequate. Therefore the achieved results are frequently temporary and the treatment palliative. Sometimes one has to watch powerless and frustrated, how, due to reproliferation, the initially successfully operated cases turn into definite failures. Thereby the extreme surgery is a double-edged sword, which during the operation can solve previously unsolvable problems but at the same time can bring new stimulation to the proliferative process.

This fact, combined with attractiveness and technical fascination of the new technique presents also the danger of the extreme surgery. Retinal surgery, transvitreal fixation with retinal tacks and silicone tamponade are powerful technical means, by which one can, practically always, achieve attachment of the retina at the end of the operation. As attachment of the retina at the end of the operation is the first aim of every surgeon, the temptation is great to use these powerful means too early or even unnecessarily and without the preparatory work. Sad results of this wrong use of retinal surgery have lately been frequently seen and sometimes, unfortunately, ascribed to the technique itself.

Summing up, one could say that the optimum surgical results are to be found in a balance between the well-considered aggressive, radical surgery and an as atraumatic as possible performance of that surgery. To realize these two demands, which are frequently difficult to combine, a preoperative assessment and an operative plan respecting relevant surgical rules are an absolute necessity.

Finally, the question arises what else can be done to further improve our results, which are not quite satisfying. As in all pathoanatomic entities coming into consideration for this surgical treatment, the problem is basically biological, and a real therapeutic breakthrough can be expected only from the pharmacological therapy. Without going deeper into this problem, it seems, unfortunately, not justified to believe that such a breakthrough is to be expected in the near future. Therefore, our attention and our efforts should be concentrated on two matters: prevention and surgical treatment. It is perhaps strange that at the end of a surgical book prevention is called to assistance, but it is certain that a great number of cases operated daily in this technique, need not have been operated if the first operation or the subsequent follow-up had been better. Better conventional surgery and particularly treatment of the endangered fellow-eye in detachment patients, better primary repair and follow-up of trauma patients, timely laser treatment of diabetics can make treatment with vitrectomy and silicone superfluous in a great number of patients.

In the near future a breakthrough in vitreoretinal surgery comparable to

172

vitrectomy and retinal surgery can hardly be expected. Improvement of the results, as it concerns mostly avoiding of reproliferation, should therefore be sought in improvement of instrumentation and in atraumatic surgery. As long as there are no dependable pharmacological means against reproliferation, a long-term tamponade will be necessary. In the near future appearance and introduction of new materials for internal tamponade, better than silicone, is to be expected. As long as these are not yet available, use of purified silicone is to be recommended, by which, perhaps, emulsification and its consequences can be avoided. Use of heavy silicone as an instrument during the operation, in certain clinical forms of PVR detachment, is also to be considered.

Anyhow, vitreoretinal surgery with silicone tamponade remains, without the support of pharmacological therapy, a technique with an uncertain outcome. It remains, however, because of its technical fascination and not rare spectacular results in the most difficult cases, a challenge for those who are prepared to tackle hard work and sometimes face disappointment.

Bibliography

Abrams G., Williams G.A., Neuwirth J., McDonald R.: Clinical results of titanium retinal tacks with pneumatic insertion. *Am. J. Ophthalmol.*, 102, 13–19, 1986.

Albert D., Alexandrides E.: Hornhaut-endothelbefunde und Silikonöl-implantation: Erste Befunde. *Fortschr. Ophthalmol.*, 82, 283–284, 1985.

Alexandrides E., Daniel H.: Results of silicone oil injection into the vitreous. *Dev. Ophthalmol.*, Karger, Basel, 2, 24–27, 1981.

Ando F., Kondo J.: A plastic tack for the treatment of retinal detachment with giant tear. *Am. J. Ophthalmol.*, 95, 260–261, 1983.

Ando F.: Intraocular hypertension resulting from pupillary block by silicone oil. *Am. J. Ophthalmol.*, 99, 87–88, 1985.

Ando F., Miyabe Y., Oshima K., Yamanaka A.: Temporary use of intraocular silicone oil in the treatment of complicated retinal detachment. *Graefe's Arch. Clin. Exp. Ophthalmol.*, 224, 32–33, 1986.

Armaly M.F.: Ocular tolerance to aqueous and vitreous replacement by silicone fluid. *Pres. at Midwestern section of the Association for Research in Ophthalmol.*, Kansas City, April, 29–30, 1961.

Armaly M.F.: Ocular tolerance to silicones I. Replacement of aqueous and vitreous by silicone fluids. *Arch. Ophthalmol.*, 68, 390–395, 1962.

Armaly M.F.: More ocular uses of silicone forms. *Invest. Ophthalmol.*, 1, 434, 1962.

Armaly M.F.: Experimental intraocular uses of silicone fluids. *Invest. Ophthalmol.*, 1, 801, 1962.

Bacin F., Gibert Ch.: Résultats du traitement des décollements de rétine avec rétraction du vitré par injection de silicone liquide intraoculaire. *Bull. Soc. Ophtalmol. Fr.*, LXXXII, 367–372, 1982.

Barthelemy F., A.L.: Utilisation de l'huile de silicone en tamponnement transitoire dans le traitement des décollements de rétine avec rétraction vitreoretinienne. I. Résultats anatomiques et fonctionnels à court et longtermes sur 110 cas. *J.Fr. Ophtalmol.*, 7, 723–777, 1984.

Beekhuis W.H., van Rij R., Zivojnović R.: Silicone oil keratopathy: Indications for keratoplasty. *Brit. J. Ophthalmol.*, 69, 247–253, 1985.

Billington B.M., Leaver P.K.: Vitrectomy and fluid-silicone exchange for giant retinal tears: Results at 18 months. *Graefe's Arch. Clin. Exp. Ophthalmol.*, 224, 7–10, 1986.

Blodi F.C.: Injection and impregnation of liquid silicone into ocular tissues. *Am. J. Ophthalmol.*, 71, 1044–1951, 1971.

Bonnét I.: Essais de traitement de certains décollements de rétine par injection de silikone intravitréen. *Bull. Soc. Ophthalmol. Fr.*, 64, 451–453, 1964.

Cairns J.D. et al.: Combined vitrectomy, intraocular micro surgery and liquid silicone in the treatment of proliferative vitreoretinopathy. *Aust. J. Ophthalmol.*, 12, 133–138, 1984.

174

Castren J.A.: Retinal detachment and intraocular silicone fluid injection. *Ann. Med. Exp. Fenn.*, 42, 1–3, 1964.

Chan C., Okun E.: The question of ocular tolerance to intravitreal liquid silicone. *Ophthalmology*, 93, 651–660, 1986.

Chauvaud D., Fraisse F., Verdière B.: A propos d'un cas d'oedème aiqu du poumon observé après insection intra oculaire d'huile de silicone. *J. Fr. Ophtalmol.*, 6, 635–637, 1983.

Chauvaud D., A.L.: Utilisation de l'huile de silicone et tamponnement transitoire dans le traitement des décollements de rétine avec rétraction vitréo-rétinienne. II aspects, prévention et traitement des complications. *J. Fr. Ophtalmol.*, 7, 279–284, 1984.

Chauvaud D.: Tamponnement interne par huile de silicone pour traitement des décollements de rétine. *J. Fr. Ophtalmol.*, 9, 251–260, 1986.

Chignell A.H.: Silicone injection. In: A.H. Chignell, *Retinal detachment surgery*. Springer Verlag, Heidelberg, 90–91, 1980.

Cibis P.A., Becker B., Okun E., Canaan S.: The use of liquid silicone in retinal detachment surgery. *Arch. Ophthalmol.*, 68, 590–599, 1962.

Cibis P.A.: Vitreous transfer and silicone injections. *Trans. Am. Acad. Ophthalmol.*, 68, 983–987, 1964.

Cibis P.A.: Recent methods in the surgical treatment of retinal detachment: Intravitreal procedures. *Trans. Ophthalmol. Soc. U.K.*, 85, 111–127, 1965.

Cibis P.A.: Vitroretinal pathology and surgery in retinal detachment. *C.V. Mosby Publishing Company*, St. Louis, 1965.

Cleary P.E.: Vitrectomy and silicone oil in ocular trauma. A preliminary report. *Int. Ophthalmol.*, 5, 114, 1982.

Clemens S., Kroll P.: Echographische Befunde nach intra-vitrealer Silikoninstillation. *Klin. Mbl. Augenheilkunde*, 185, 17–21, 1984.

Clemens S., Kroll P.: Ultrasonic findings after treatment of retinal detachment by intravitreal silicone instillation. *Am. J. Ophthalmol.*, 98, 369–373, 1984.

Cockerham W.D., Schepens C.L., Freeman H.M.: Silicone injection in retinal detachment. *Mod. Probl. Ophthalmol.*, Karger, Basel, 8, 525–540, 1969.

Cockerham W., Schepens C.L., Freeman H.M.: Silicone injection in retinal detachment. *Arch. Ophthalmol.*, 83, 704–712, 1970.

Cockerham W.D., Schepens C.L., MacKenzie Freeman H.M.: Silicone injection in retinal detachment. *Arch. Ophthalmol.*, (Chicago) 83, 395–404, 1976.

Cohen S.B., Peyman G.A., de Corral L.R.: Extracapsular cataractextraction after silicone oil injection (letter). *Ophthalmol. Surg.*, 16, 660, 1985.

Constable I., Mohamed S., Tan P.L.: Superviscous silicone liquid in retinal surgery. *Austr. J. Ophthalmol.*, 10, 5–11, 1982.

de Corral L.R., Peyman G.A.: Silicone oil injection in aphakic eyes: A modified technique. *Ophthalmol. Surg.*, 16, 774–775, 1985.

Cox M.S., Trese M.T., Murphy P.L.: Silicone oil for advanced proliferative vitreoretinopathy. *Ophthalmology*, 93, 646–650, 1986.

Crips A., de Juan E. Jr., Tiedeman J.: Effect of silicone oil viscosity on emulsification. *Arch. Ophthalmol.*, 1987, in press.

McCuen B., Landers M.B., Machemer R.: The use of silicone oil following failed vitrectomy for retinal detachment with advanced proliferative vitreoretinopathy. *Ophthalmology*, 92, 1029–1034, 1985.

McCuen B., Landers M.B., Machemer R.: The use of silicone oil following failed vitrectomy for retinal detachment with advanced proliferative vitreoretinopathy. *Graefe's Arch. Clin. Exp. Ophthalmol.*, 224, 38–39, 1986.

McCuen B., de Jùan E., Machemer R.: Silicone oil in vitreoretinal surgery part I: Surgical techniques. *Retina*, 5, 189–197, 1985.

McCuen B., de Juan E., Landers M.B., Machemer R.: Silicone oil in vitreorétinal surgery part II: Results and complications. *Retina,* 5, 198–205, 1985.

Deutman A.F., Eijkenboom G.J.M., Fanuriakis C.: A microsurgical method for the injection of intraocular silicone oil. *Int. Ophthalmol.,* 2, 63–69, 1980.

Diddie K., Fastenberg D., Delmage J., Dorey K.: The effect of intraocular silicone oil in experimental massive periretinal proliferation. *Int. Ophthalmol.,* 5, 119, 1982.

Dimopoulos S.: Silikonöl Injektion in der Netzhaut – Glaskörperchirurgie. Inaugural Disertation zur Erlangung der Doktorwürde der hohen Medizinischen Fakultät der Universität Köln, 1–2, 1985.

Dimopoulos S., Heimann K.: Spätkomplikationen nach Silikonölinjektion. Langzeitbeobachtungen an 100 Fällen. *Klin. Mbl. Augenheilkunde,* 189, 223–227, 1986.

Dodd C.L.: Preretinal retraction. Silicone oil injection. *Trans Ophthalmol. Soc. U.K.,* 99, 43–44, 1979.

Dufour R.: L'injection intra-vitréenne de silicone liquide dans le décollement rétinien désespéré. *Ophthalmologica (Basel),* 147, 160–166, 1964.

Dufour R.: Experience with intraocular silicone injection. In: A. McPherson, *New and controversial aspects of retinal detachment.* New York Hoeber Med. Div., Harper and Row, 377–382, 1968.

Eckardt C., Martin H., Utermann D.: Zur Endochirurgie subretinalen Stränge bei proliferative Vitreoretinopathie. *Klin. Mbl. Augenheilkunde,* 187, 21–24, 1985.

Eckardt C., Utermann D.: Chirurgische Pupillenerweiterung in Rahmen komplizierter Amotio operationen. *Klin. Mbl. Augenheilkunde,* 188, 118–121, 1986.

Esser J., Foerster M.H., Laqua H.: ERG-befunde bei Patienten mit intraoculärer Silikonöl-füllung. *Fortschr. Ophthalmol.,* 80, 128–129, 1983.

Failer J., Faulborn J., Erb P.: Die Phagocystose von Silikonölen unterschiedlicher Viskosität durch peritoneal Makrophagen der Maus. *Klin. Mbl. Augenheilkunde,* 184, 450–452, 1984.

Fastenberg D.M., Diddie K.R., Delmage J.M., Dorey K.: Intraocular injection of silicone oil for experimental proliferative vitreoretinopathy. *Am. J. Ophthalmol.,* 95, 663–667, 1983.

Faulborn J.: Indikation für Silikonöl-implantation bei fortgeschrittener proliferativer diabetischer Retinopathie. *Klin. Mbl. Augenheilkunde,* 185, 362–363, 1984.

Faulborn J., Bowald S.: Silikonöl in epiretinalen Membranen 3–4 Monate nach Implantation: Mikroskopische Befunde in 2 Fällen. *Klin. Mbl. Augenheilkunde,* 188, 133–134, 1986.

Feltesse-Koegler M.C.: Etude de 300 cas de décollements de rétine opérés par la technique vitrectomie tamponnement interne par l'huile de silicone. Thèse Médecine, Paris XIII, 225 p., 1983.

Foerster M.H., Esser J., Laqua H.: Silicone oil and its influence on electrophysiologic findings. *Am. J. Ophthalmol.,* 99, 201–206, 1985.

François P., Khoury J., Blervacques A.: Décollement de rétine et silicone. *Bull. Soc. Ophthalmol. Fr.,* LXX, 593–602, 1970.

Frumar K.D., Gregor Z.J., Carter R.M., Arden G.B.: Electrophysiological responses after vitrectomy and intraocular tamponade. *Trans. Ophthalmol. Soc. U.K.,* 104, 129–132, 1985.

Gabel V.P., Kampik A., Gabel Ch., Spiegel D.: Silicone oil with high specific gravity for intraocular use. *Brit. J. Ophthalmol.,* 71, –148, April 1987.

Gabel V.P., Kampik A., Burkhardt J.: Analysis of silicone oil for intraocular use of various origins. Will be published in *Graefe's Arch. of Ophthalmol.*

Gavin O., Cohentervaert D., Lean J.S.: Aqueous concentration of fluorouracil after intravitreal injection. Normal vitrectomized and silicone-filled eyes. *Arch. Ophthalmol.,* 104, 431–434, 1986.

Glaser B., Bustros S., Michels R.: Postoperative retinal breaks occurring after intravitreal silicone oil injection. *Retina,* 4, 246–248, 1984.

176

Gnad H. et al.: Silikonölimplantation – erste Erfahrungen mit einer modifizierten Technik. *Klin. Mbl. Augenheilkunde,* 183, 384–386, 1983.

Gnad H., Skorpik Ch., Paroussis P.: Funktionelle und anatomische Resultate nach temporärer Silikonöl-implantation. *Klin. Mbl. Augenheilkunde,* 185, 364–367, 1984.

Gnad H., Paroussis P., Skorpik C.: An intraocular balloon for silicone oil implantation. *Graefe's Arch. Clin. Exp. Ophthalmol.,* 224, 18–20, 1986.

Gonvers M.: Usage temporaire de silicone intra-oculaire dans le traitement des décollements de rétine avec prolifération périrétinienne massive. *Klin. Mbl. Augenheilkunde,* 180, 382–384, 1982.

Gonvers M.: Temporary use of intraocular silicone oil in the treatment of detachment with massive preretinal proliferation. Preliminary report. *Ophthalmologica,* Basel, 184, 210–218, 1982.

Gonvers M.: Temporary use of intraocular silicone oil in the treatment of retinal detachment with massive periretinal retraction. *Int. Ophthalmol.,* 5, 86, 1982.

Gonvers M.: Temporary use of silicone oil in the treatment of special cases of retinal detachment. *Ophthalmologica,* 187, 202–209, 1983.

Gonvers M., Tresher R.: Temporary use of silicone oil in the treatment of proliferative vitreo-retinopathy. An experimental study with a new animal model. *Graefe's Arch. Ophthalmol.,* 221, 46–53, 1983.

Gonvers M.: Silikonöl und proliferative Vitreo-retinopathie. Eine experimentele Studie. *Klin. Mbl. Augenheilkunde,* 184, 449, 1984.

Gonvers M.: A new silicone oil pump (letter). *Am. J. Ophthalmol.,* 99, 210, 1985.

Gonvers M.: Temporary silicone oil tamponade in the management of retinal detachment with proliferative vitreoretinopathy. *Am. J. Ophthalmol.,* 100, 239–245, 1985.

Gonvers M., Hornung J.P., de Courten Ch.: The effect of liquid silicone on the rabbit retina. *Arch. Ophthalmol.,* 104, 1057–1062, 1986.

Gonvers M.: Vorübergehende Tamponade mit Silikonöl in der Behandlung der proliferativen Vitreoretinopathie: 5 Jahre Erfahrung. *Klin. Mbl. Augenheilkunde,* 188, 405, 1986.

Grey R.H.B., Leaver P.K.: Results of silicone oil injection in massive preretinal retraction. *Trans. Ophthalmol., Soc. U.K.,* 97, 238–241, 1977.

Grey R.H.B., Leaver P.K.: Silicone oil in the treatment of massive preretinal retraction I. Results in 105 eyes. *Brit. J. Ophthalmol.,* 63, 355–360, 1979.

Grey R.H.B., Leaver P.K.: Silicone oil in treatment of preretinal retraction. *Trans. Ophthalmol. Soc. U.K.,* 97, 238–241, 1979.

Grisolono J., Peyman G.: Special short needle to inject and aspirate high viscosity silicone oil. Arch. Ophthalmol., 104, 608, 1986.

Haut J., Ullern M., Boulard M.L., Cedah A.: Utilisation du silicone intra-oculaire après vitrectomie comme traitement des rétractions massive du vitré (Note préliminaire). *Bull. Soc. Ophtalmol. Fr.,* 78, 361–365, 1978.

Haut J., Ullern M., Chatellier Ph., Cedah A.: Résultats de 200 cas d'injection intra-oculaire de silicone associée à la vitrectomie. *Bull. Mem. Soc. Fr. Ophtalmol.,* 91, 180–184, 1979.

Haut J., Ullern M., Chermet M., van Effenterre G.: Complications des injections intra-oculaires de silicone. *Bull. Soc. Ophtalmol. Fr.,* LXXX, 519–523, 1980.

Haut J., van Effenterre G., Ullern M., Chermet M.: Traitement chirurgical des décollements de rétine avec trou maculaire par la technique de la vitrectomie associée à l'injection de silicone liquide. *J. Fr. Ophtalmol.* 3, 115–118, 1980.

Haut J., Ullern M., Chermet M., van Effenterre G.: Complications of intraocular injections of silicone combined with vitrectomy. *Ophthalmologica (Basel),* 180, 29–35, 1980.

Haut J., Chermet M., van Effenterre G., Robert P.: Technique et résultats de l'injection de silicone liquide à la vitrectomie dans le traitement des inversions rétiniennes. *Bull. Soc. Ophtalmol. Fr.,* LXXX, 517–518, 1980.

Haut J., Ullern M., Biehler D.: Problèmes par la présence et l'absence du cristallin dans les injections intra-oculaires de silicone. *Bull. Soc. Ophtalmol. Fr.*, LXXXI, 909–912, 1981.

Haut J., Larricart P., Sfeir T., van Effenterre G.: Treatment of epiretinal membranes: Report of 40 operated cases. *Ophthalmoligica*, 183, 190–196, 1981.

Haut J., Ullern M., van Effenterre G., Chermet M.: Utilisation du silicone intra-oculaire à propos de 200 cas. *Bull. Soc. Ophtalmol. Fr.*, 79, 797–799, 1981.

Haut J., Leon M.C., van Effenterre G., Monin Cl., Sfeir T.: Traitement en première intention de certains décollements de rétine à rétine souple (trou maculaire, déchirure géante) par la technique de vitrectomie-silicone. *Bull. Soc. Ophtalmol. Fr.*, LXXXII, 305–309, 1982.

Haut J., Larricart P., Flamand M.: Indications of limited retinectomies in the treatment of retinal detachment and its prevention. *Int. Ophthalmol.*, 5, 118, 1982.

Haut J., van Effenterre G., Flamand M.: Treatment of retinal detachment due to macular hole using silicone oil with or without complementary argo laser photocoagulation. *Ophthalmologica (Basel)*, 87, 25–28, 1983.

Haut J.: L'intervention vitrectomie-silicone, à propos de 1.000 cas. Masson, 1984.

Haut J., Larricart P., van Effenterre G., Pinon-Pignero Fl.: Some of the most important properties of silicone oil to explain its action. *Ophthalmologica*, 191, 150–153, 1985.

Haut J., Larricart P., Geant G., van Effenterre G., Vachet J.M.: Circular subtotal retinectomy and inferior semicircular retinotomy. *Ophthalmologica*, 192, 129–134, 1986.

Heimann K., Dimopoulos S., Paulmann H.: Silikonöl Injektion in der Behandlung komplizierten Netzhautablösungen. *Klin. Mbl. Augenheilkunde*, 185, 505–508, 1984.

Heimann K., Dimopoulos S.: Intra- und postoperative Komplikationen bei silikonölinjektion zur Behandlung komplizierte Netzhautablösungen. *Klin. Mbl. Augenheilkunde*, 185, 371–372, 1984.

Heimann K., Dimopoulos S.: Die Behandlung der komplizierten Netzhautablösungen bei Pseudophakie (summary). *Klin. Mbl. Augenheilkunde*, 186, 321, 1985.

Höpping W.: Lichtkoagulation nach Glaskörperersatz durch Silikon. *Ber. Dtsch. Ophthalmol. Ges.*, 66, 336–343, 1964.

de Juan E., Hicking Bottam D., Machemer R.: Retinal tacks. *Am. J. Ophthalmol.*, 99, 272–274, 1985.

de Juan E., McCuen B., Tiedeman J.: Intraocular tamponade and surface tension. *Surv. Ophthalmol.*, 30, 47–51, 1985.

de Juan E., Hardy M., Hatchell D.L., Hatchell M.C.: The effect of intraocular silicone oil on anterior chamber oxygenpressure in cats. *Arch. Ophthalmol.*, 104, 1063–1064, 1986.

Kampik A., Gabel V.P., Spiegel D.: Tamponade mit hochviskösem Silikonöl bei massiver proliferativer Vitreo-retinopathie. *Klin. Mbl. Augenheilkunde*, 185, 368–370, 1984.

Kampik A.: Silicone oil interaction with ocular tissue. *Graefe's Arch. Clin. Exp. Ophthalmol.*, 1987, in press.

Kanski J.J., Daniel R.: Intravitreal silicone injection in retinal detachment. *Brit. J. Ophthalmol.*, 57, 542–545, 1973.

Karel I., Filipse M., Vrabec F., Obenberger J.: The effect of liquid silicone on the corneal endothelium in rabbits. *Graefe's Arch. Clin. Exp. Ophthalmol.*, 224, 481–485, 1986.

Kirchof B., Tavakolian U., Paulmann H., Heimann K.: Histopathological findings in eyes after silicone oil injection. *Graefe's Arch. Clin. Exp. Ophthalmol.*, 224, 34–37, 1986.

Kroll P., Busse A., Berg P., Clemens S.: Intraokuläre Therapie maculalochbedingte Netzhautveränderungen. *Klin. Mbl. Augenheilkunde*, 187, 499–502, 1985.

Kroll P., Hennekes R., Berg P.: Linsentrübungen nach intravitrealen Silikoninjektion. *Fortschr. Ophthalmol.*, 82, 235–236, 1985.

Labelle P., Okun E.: Ocular tolerance to liquid silicone: An experimental study. *Can. J. Ophthalmol.*, 7, 199–204, 1972.

178

Laqua H., Machemer R.: Glia cell proliferation in retinal detachment / Massive periretinal proliferation. *Am. J. Ophthalmol.*, 80, 602–618, 1975.

Laqua H., Herwig M., Wessing A., Meyer-Schwickerath G.: Silikonöl-injektion zur Behandlung komplizierter Netzhautablösungen. *Fortschr. Ophthalmol.*, 79, 233–235, 1982.

Laqua H.: Die Behandlung der Ablatio mit Makulaforamen nach der Methode von Gonvers und Machemer. *Klin. Mbl. Augenheilkunde*, 186, 13–17, 1985.

Laroche L., Pavlakis C., Saraux H., Orcel L.: Ocular findings following intravitreal silicone injection. *Arch. Ophthalmol.*, 101, 1422–1425, 1983.

Launay F., Laroche G., Limon S.: Modifications de la réfraction après injections intra-oculaires de silicone liquide. *J. Fr. Ophtalmol.*, 5, 417–425, 1982.

Lean J.S., van der Zee A.M., Ryan S.J.: Experimental model of proliferative vitreoretinopathy in the vitrectomized eye. Effect of silicone oil. *Brit. J. Ophthalmol.*, 68, 332–335, 1984.

Lean J.S., Leaver P.K., Cooling R.J., McLeod D.: Management of complex retinal detachment by vitrectomy and fluid silicone exchange. *Trans. Ophthalmol. Soc. U.K.*, 102, 203–205, 1982.

Lean J.S., Cooling R.J.: The management of post traumatic complex retinal detachment by pars plana vitrectomy and fluid silicone exchange. *Int. Ophthalmol.*, 5, 114, 1982.

Leaver P.K.: Silicone oil injection in the treatment of massive preretinal retraction. In: A. McPherson, New and controversial aspects of vitreoretinal surgery. C.V. Mosby Co., St. Louis, 397–401, 1977.

Leaver P.K., Garner A., Grey R.H.B., Hitchings R.A.: Effects of intraocular silicone. *Trans. Ophthalmol. Soc. U.K.*, 97, 633, 1977.

Leaver P.K., Grey R.H., Garner A.: Complications following silicone oil injection. *Mod. Probl. Ophthalmol.*, 20, 290–294, 1979.

Leaver P.K., Grey R.H., Garner A.: Silicone oil injection in the treatment of massive preretinal retraction. II. Late complications in 93 eyes. *Brit. J. Ophthalmol.*, 63, 361–367, 1979.

Leaver P.K., Grey R.H.B., Garner A.: Complications following silicone oil injection. *Mod. Probl. Ophthalmol.*, Karger, Basel, 20, 290–294, 1979.

Leaver P.K., Grey R.H., Garner R.: Silicone oil injection in the treatment of massive preretinal retraction. II. Late complications in 93 eyes. *Brit. J. Ophthalmol.*, 63, 361–367, 1979.

Leaver P.K., Lean J.S.: Management of giant retinal tears using vitrectomy and silicone oil/fluid exchange. *Trans. Ophthalmol. Soc. U.K.*, 101, 189–191, 1981.

Leaver P.K., Lean J.S.: Results and complications of silicone oil injection in the treatment of massive preretinal proliferation. *Int. Ophthalmol.*, 5, 86, 1982.

Leaver P.K., Cooling R.J., Feretis E.: Vitrectomy and fluid silicone exchange for giant retinal tears results at six months. *Brit. J. Ophthalmol.*, 68, 432–438, 1984.

Leaver P.K.: Long-standing retinal-detachments the role of internal tamponade. *Trans. Ophthalmol. Soc. U.K.*, 105, 476–479, 1986.

Lee P.F., Donovan R.M., Mukai N., Schepens C.L., Freeman H.: Intravitreous injection of silicone. An experimental study. I. Clinical picture and histology of the eye. *Ann. Ophthalmol.*, 1, 15–25, 1969.

Lemmen K.D., Michel K., Kirchof B., Paulmann H., Heimann K.: Klinische und morphologische Aspekte der Silikonölkeratopathie in Tierexperiment. *Fortschr. Ophthalmol.* 82, 556–558, 1985.

McLeod D.: Silicone oil injection during closed microsurgery for diabetic retinal detachment. *Graefe's Arch. Clin. Exp. Ophthalmol.*, 224, 55–59, 1986.

Leon M.C.: Traitement de certains décollements de la rétina avec rétine souple par la technique de vitrectomie-silicone (à propos de 29 cas). Thèse doct. Med., Paris, 37 p., 1981.

Levine A.M., Ellis R.A.: Intraocular liquid silicone implants. *Am. J. Ophthalmol.*, 55, 939–943, 1963.

Liesenhoff H.: Ueber eine verbesserte Technik bei der Silikon-injektion in den Glasköperraum während der Ablatio-Operation. *Klin. Mbl. Augenheilkunde*, 125, 658–665, 1968.

Liesenhoff H., Schmitt J.: Komplikationen durch flüssiges Silikon in der Vorderkammer. *Ber. Dtsch. Ophthalmol. Ges.*, 69, 643–644, 1969.

Limon S., Offret H., Sourdille Ph.: La dissection de la membrane épirétinienne au silicone. In: Chirurgie du vitré. *Bull. Soc. Ophtalmol. Fr.*, Rapport annuel, 208–232, 1978.

Limon S., Laroche G., Launay F.: Modifications de la réfraction après injections intra-oculaires de silicone liquide. *J.Fr. Ophtalmol.*, 5, 417–425, 1982.

Lund O.E.: Silikon als Glaskörperersatz. *Ber. Dtsch. Ophthalmol. Ges.*, 68, 166–169, 1968.

Machemer R.: Pigment epithelium proliferation in retinal detachment: (massive periretinal proliferation). *Am. J. Ophthalmol.*, 80, 1–23, 1975.

Machemer R.: Massive periretinal proliferation a logical approach to therapy. *Trans. Am. Ophthalmol. Soc.*, 75, 556–586, 1977.

Machemer R.: Pathogenesis and classification of massive preretinal proliferation. *Brit. J. Ophthalmol.*, 62, 737–747, 1978.

Machemer R., Laqua H.: A logical approach to the treatment of massive preretinal proliferation. *Ophthalmology*, 85, 584–593, 1978.

Machemer R.: Schneiden der Netzhaut: Eine Behandlungsmöglichkeit zum Wiederanlegen der Netzhaut. *Klin. Mbl. Augenheilkunde*, 175, 597–601, 1979.

Machemer R.: Surgical approaches to subretinal strands. *Am. J. Ophthalmol.*, 90, 81–85, 1980.

Machemer R.: Retinotomy. *Am. J. Ophthalmol.*, 92, 768–774, 1981.

Machemer R.: The importance of fluid absorption, traction, intraocular currents, and chorioretinal scars in the therapy of rhegmatogenous retinal detachments. XLI Edward Jackson Memorial Lecture. *Am. J. Ophthalmol.*, 98, 681–693, 1984.

Manschot W.A.: Intravitreal silicone injection. *Adv. Ophthalmol.*, Karger, Basel, 36, 197–207, 1978.

Martola E.L., Dohlman C.H.: Silicone oil in the anterior chamber of the eye. *Acta Ophthalmol. (Köln)*, 41, 75–79, 1963.

Meredith T.A., Lindsey D.T., Goldman A.I.: E.R.G. evaluation after vitrectomy and silicone oil injection. *ARVO, (Supp. Invest. Ophthalmol. Visual Sci.)*, 199, 1981.

Meredith T.A., Lindsey D.T.: Electroretinographic studies following vitrectomy and intraocular silicone oil injection. *Brit. J. Ophthalmol.*, 69, 254–260, 1985.

Mester U., Rothe R., Zubcov A.: Experimental studies with high density silicone oil for giant retinal tear. *Ophthalmol. Res.*, 18, 81–86, 1986.

Meyer-Schwickerath G.R.E., Lund O.O., Höpping W.: Six years' experience with silicone injections into the vitreous cavity. In: *Symposium on retina and retinal surgery*. C.V. Mosby, St. Louis, 239, 1969.

Miyamoto K., Refoso M.F., Tolentino F.I., Fournier G.A., Albert D.M.: Fluorinated oils as experimental vitreous substitutes. *Arch. Ophthalmol.*, 104, 1033–1056, 1986.

Momirov D., van Lith G.H.M., Zivojnović R.: E.R.G. and E.O.G. of eyes with intravitreously injected silicone oil. *Ophthalmologica*, 186, 183–188, 1983.

Moreau P.G.: Implant into the vitreous using silicone for detachment of the retina. *Trans. Ophthalmol. Soc. U.K.*, 84, 167–171, 1964.

Moreau P.G.: Premiers essais d'injections de silicones liquides intraoculaires dans le décollement de la rétine. *Bull. Soc. Ophtalmol. Fr.*, 64, 130–133, 1964.

Moreau P.G.: Les injections de silicones liquides dans le décollement de la rétine. *Bull. Soc. Ophtalmol. Fr.*, 79, 488–496, 1966.

Moreau P.G.: Les silicones intraoculaires dans les décollements de rétine désespérés. *Ann. Oculist.*, 200, 257–265, 1967.

Mukai N., Lee P.F., Schepens G.L.: Intravitreous injection of silicone an experimental study II. Histochemistry and electron microscopy. *Ann. Ophthalmol.*, 4, 273–287, 1972.

Mukai N., Lee P.F., Oguri M., Schepens G.L.: A long-term evaluation of silicone retinopathy in monkeys. *Can. J. Ophthalmol.*, 10, 391–402, 1975.

Nauman G.O.H., Kleinknecht K.: Silikonsausräumung aus der Vorderkammer. *Ber. Dtsch. Ophthalmol. Ges.*, 75, 625, 1977.

Ni C., Wang W.J., Albert D.M. et al.: Intravitreous siliconinjection histopathological findings in a human eye after 12 years. *Arch. Ophthalmol.*, 101, 1399–1401, 1983.

Niesel P., Fankhauser F.: Zur retrovitrealen Silikoninjektion bei der Behandlung der Netzhautablösung. *Ophthalmologica (Basel)*, 147, 167–175, 1964.

Ober R., Blanko J., Ogden T., Minckler D., Ryan S.: Retinal tolerance to liquid silicone: An experimental study. *Int. Ophthalmol.*, 5, 118, 1982.

Ober R., Blanks J.C., Ogden T.E. et al.: Experimental retinal tolerance to liquid silicone. *Retina*, 3, 77–84, 1985.

Okun E.: Die Behandlung der durch massive praeretinale Fibroplasie komplizierte Netzhautablösung. *Ber. Dtsch. Ophthalmol. Ges.*, LXVIII, 145–149, 1967.

Okun E.: Intravitreal surgery utilizing liquid silicone. A long-term follow-up. *Trans. Pacif. Cst. Otoophthalmol. Soc.*, 49, 141–159, 1968.

Okun E.: Therapy of retinal detachment complicated by massive preretinal fibrosis. Ber. Dtsch. Ophthalmol. Ges., 68, 145–150, 1968.

Okun E., Arribas N.P.: Therapy of retinal detachment complicated by massive preretinal fibroplasia: Long-term follow-up of patients treated with intravitreal silicone. *Trans. New Orleans Acad. Ophthalmol.*, 278–293, 1969.

Okun E.: The current status of silicone oil. Analysis of long-term successes. In: A.V. Irvine, C. O'Malley, eds., *Advances in Vitreous Surgery*, Charlos C. Thomas, Springfield, Illinois, 47, 518–522, 1976.

Parnley V.C., Barishak Y.R., Howes E.L., Crawfórd B.: Foreign body giant cell reaction to liquid silicone. *Am. J. Ophthalmol.*, 101, 680–683, 1986.

Paulmann H.: Sekundäre Versorgung in hinteren Abschnitt. *Fortschr. Ophthalmol.*, 81, 543–547, 1984.

Paylor R.P., Peyman G.: A method to locate the silicone oil aqueous humor interface (correspondence). *Arch. Ophthalmol.*, 103, 1782–1783, 1985.

Petersen J., Ritzau-Tondrow U., Vogel M.: Fluor-Silikonöl schwerer als Wasser: ein neues Hilfmittel der vitreo-retinal Chirurgie. *Klin. Mbl. Augenheilkunde*, 189, 228–232, 1986.

Peyman G., Ericson E., May D.: A review of substances and techniques of vitreous replacement. *Survey Ophthalmol.*, 17, 41–51, 1972.

Peyman G., de Corral L.: One step extracapsular extraction and silicone oil injection in the management of proliferative vitreoretinopathy. *Brit. J. Ophthalmol.*, 70, 382–386, 1986.

Polemann G., Froitzheim G.: Tierexperimentelle Untersuchungen zur biologischen Verträglichkeit von Silikonen. *Arzneimittel-Forschung*, 3, 457, 1953.

Poujol J., Haut J., Fleury P.: Corrections â apporter dans l'examen échographique des yeux remplis de silicone liquide. *Bull. Soc. Ophtalmol. Fr.*, LXXVIII, 367–369, 1978.

Ravault M., Trepsat C.: Le silicone intra-oculaire dans le traitement du décollement de la rétine. Indications, notes techniques. *Bull. Soc. Ophtalmol. Fr.*, LXXXI, 509–510, 1981.

Refojo M.F., Roldan M., Leong F., Henriquez A.S.: Effect of silicone oil on the cornea. *J. Biomed. Mat. Ses.*, 19, 643–652, 1985.

Rentsch F.J., Atzler P., Liesenhoff H.: Histologische und elektronmikroskopische Untersuchungen an einem menschlichen Auge nach mehrjährige intravitrealer Silikonimplantation. *Ber. Dtsch. Ophthalmol. Ges.*, 75, 70–74, 1977.

The Retina Society Terminology Committee: The classification of retinal detachment with proliferative vitreoretinopathy. *Ophthalmology*, 90, 121–125, 1983.

Rinkoff J.S., de Juan E., McCuen B.: Silicone oil for retinal detachment with advanced proliferative vitreoretinopathy following failed vitrectomy for proliferative diabetic retinopathy. *Am. J. Ophthalmol.*, 101, 181–186, 1986.

Rosengren B.: Intravitreous injection of liquid silicone for retinal detachment. Transections Swedish Ophthalmol. Society. *Acta Ophthalmol.*, 44, 975–976, 1966.

Rosengren B.: Silicone into the vitreous in hopeless cases of retinal detachment. *Acta Ophthalmol.*, (Kbn), 47, 757–760, 1969.

Roussat B., Ruellan Y.M.: Traitement du décollement de la rétine par vitrectomie et injection d'huile de silicone. Résultats à long terme et complications de 105 cas. *J. Fr. Ophtalmol.*, 7, 11–18, 1984.

Ruellan Y.M., Roussat B.: Décollement de rétine: Tamponnement interne provisoire par huile de silicone après vitrectomie. *J. Fr. Ophtalmol.*, 8, 117–124, 1985.

Ryan S.: The pathophysiology of proliferative vitreoretinopathy and its management. *Am. J. Ophthalmol.*, 100, 188–193, 1985.

Schepens C.L., Regan C.D.J.: Controversial aspects of the management of retinal detachment. Boston, Discussion, 191–204, 1965.

Schepens C.L.: Discussion chapitre IV. Part II sur l'injection de silicone fluide. *Mod. Probl. Ophthalmol.*, Karger, Basel, 15, 297, 1975.

Schepens C.L.: Vitreous replacement. In: Schepens C.L., *Retinal detachment and allied diseases.* W.B. Saunders Co., Phil., 2, 747–769, 1983.

Scott J.D.: Treatment of the detached immobile retina. *Trans. Ophthalmol. Soc. U.K.*, 92, 351–357, 1972.

Scott J.D.: The treatment of massive vitreous retraction. *Trans. Ophthalmol. Soc. U.K.*, 93, 417–423, 1973.

Scott J.D.: Macula holes and retinal detachment. *Trans. Ophthalmol. Soc. U.K.*, 94, 319–324, 1974.

Scott J.D.: Treatment of the detached immobile retina. *Trans. Ophthalmol. Soc. U.K.*, 92, 351–357, 1972.

Scott J.D.: The treatment of massive vitreous retraction by the separation of pre-retinal membranes using liquid silicone. *Mod. Probl. Ophthalmol.*, Karger, Basel, 15, 285, 1975.

Scott J.D.: Giant tear of the retina. *Trans. Ophthalmol. Soc. U.K.*, 95, 142–144, 1975.

Scott J.D.: Treatment of massive vitreous retraction. *Trans. Ophthalmol. Soc. U.K.*, 95, 429–432, 1975.

Scott J.D.: The treatment of massive vitreous retraction with the separation of preretinal membranes using silicone oil. In: A.R. Irvine, C. O'Malley, *Advances in vitreous surgery.* Charles C. Thomas, Springfield Ill., 523–525, 1976.

Scott J.D.: Utilisation du silicone dans la chirurgie endoculaire. *La clinique ophtalmol.*, 3, 9–18, 1977.

Scott J.D.: A rationale for the use of liquid silicone. *Trans. Ophthalmol. Soc. U.K.*, 97, 235–237, 1977.

Scott J.D.: The use and abuses of liquid silicone. In: A.F. Deutman, ed., *Documenta Ophthalmologica Proceedings Series.* Dr. W. Junk Publishers, The Hague, 7, 113–119, 1978.

Scott J.D.: A rationale for the use of liquid silicone in retinal detachment surgery. *Excerpta Med. I.C.S.*, 1/450, 433–437, 1979.

Scott J.D.: Lens changes in retinal detachment. *Trans. Ophthalmol. Soc. U.K.*, 99, 241–243, 1979.

Scott J.D.: Use of liquid silicone in vitrectomized eyes. *Dev. Ophthalmol.*, 2, 185–190, 1981.

Scott J.D.: The use of viscoelastic materials in the posterior segment. *Trans. Ophthalmol. Soc. U.K.*, 103, 280–283, 1983.

Shea M.: The use of silicone in retinal detachment surgery. *Trans. Can. Ophthalmol. Soc.*, 26, 63–78, 1963.

Shugar J.K., de Juan E., McCuen B., Tiedeman J., Landers M.R., Machemer R.: Ultrasonic examination of the silicone-filled eyes: Theoretical and practical considerations. *Graefe's Arch. Clin. Exp. Ophthalmol.*, 224, 361–367, 1986.

The Silicone Study Group: Proliferative vitreoretinopathy. *Am. J. Ophthalmol.*, 99, 593–595, 1985.

Sourdille Ph., Colin J., Baikoff G., Renard G.: Vitrectomie-injection de silicone dans un syndrome Deterson. *Bull. Soc. Ophtalmol. Fr.*, LXXX, 419–420, 1980.

Sternberg P., Hatchell D., Foulks G.A., Landers M.: The effect of silicone oil on the cornea. *Arch. Ophthalmol.*, 103, 90–91, 1985.

Stone W. Jr.: Alloplasty in surgery of the eye. *N. Engl. J. Med.*, 258, 486–490, 1958.

Sugar H.S., Okamura I.D.: Ocular findings six years after intravitreal silicone injection. *Arch. Ophthalmol. Chicago*, 94, 612–615, 1976.

Tavakolian U., Seiler T., Wollensak J.: Zur Amotio insanata. Bericht über 100 Silikonölinjektionen (Summary). *Klin. Mbl. Augenheilkunde*, 186, 398, 1985.

Tavakolian U., Heimann K., Lemmen K.D.: Zur Behandlung von Netzhautablösungen mit zentralen Foramina bei hoher Myopie. *Fortschr. Ophthalmol.*, 82, 553–555, 1985.

Tavakolian U., Wollensak J.: Komplikationen nach Silikonölinjektionen (Summary). *Klin. Mbl. Augenheilkunde*, 187, 556, 1985.

Unosson K., Stenkula S., Tornquist L., Veijdegard L.: Liquid silicone in the treatment of retinal detachment. *Acta Ophthalmol.*, 63, 656–660, 1985.

Urayama A., Sakuragi S., Takahashi N., Sakai F., Tanaka J.: A long-term follow-up to silicone retinopiesis for retinal detachment. *Jap. J. Clin. Ophthalmol.*, 28, 115, 1974.

Usui M., Hamazaki S., Takan S., Matsuo H.: A new surgical technique for the treatment of giant tears: Transvitreal fixation. *Jap. J. Ophthalmol. V.*, 23, 206–215, 1979.

Waring G.O.: Posterior collagenous layer (correspondence). *Arch. Ophthalmol.*, 103, 1278, 1985.

Watzke R.C.: Silicone retinopiesis for retinal detachment. A long-term clinical evaluation. *Arch. Ophthalmol.*, 77, 185–196, 1967.

Watzke R.C.: Silicone retinopiesis for retinal detachment. A pathologic report. *Surv. Ophthalmol.*, 12, 333–337, 1967.

Watzke R.C.: Use of silicone oil. *Arch. Ophthalmol.*, 100, 1354–1355, 1982.

Weidemann P., Heimann K.: Proliferative vitreoretinopathie. *Klin. Mbl. Augenheilkunde*, 188, 559–564, 1986.

Wessing A., Fried M.: Massive preretinale proliferation and injection of liquid silicone. In: Y. Mitsui, Ophthalmology update, (XXIII Int. Congress Opthalmol., Kyoto, 1978). Except. Med., Amsterdam, 178, 1980.

Wessing A., Laqua H., Herwig M., Meyer-Schwickerath G.: Silikonölinjektionen bei komplizierten Netzhautablösungen. *Sitzungsberichte der 140. Versammlung des Vereins. Rheinisch-Westfälischer Augenärzte*, 1981.

Živojnović R., Mertens D.A.E., Baarsma G.S.: Das flüssige Silikon in der Amotiochirurgie. Bericht über 90 Fälle. *Klin. Mbl. Augenheilkunde*, 179, 17–23, 1981.

Živojnović R., Mertens D.A.E., Peperkamp E.: Das flüssige Silikon in der Amotiochirurgie (II). Bericht über 280 Fälle – weitere Entwicklung der Technik. *Klin. Mbl. Augenheilkunde*, 181, 444–452, 1982.

Živojnović R.: Behandlung komplizierter Netzhautablösungen mit intraokulärer Silikonölinjektion. *Klin. Mbl. Augenheilkunde*, 181 (Abst.), 1982.

Živojnović R.: Rupture u makuli: Ablacija mrežnjače – tretman silikonskim uljem. *Anali Klin. Bolnice 'Dr. M. Stojanović'*, 22, 107, 1983.

Živojnović R., Vijfvinkel G.J.: A modified flute needle. *Am. J. Ophthalmol.* (letter), 1983.

Živojnović R.: Das Silikonöl in der Amotiochirurgie – neue Möglichkeiten bei der Behandlung der schwierigsten Netzhautablösungen. *Klin. Mbl. Augenheilkunde*, 185 (Abst.), 1984.

GPSR Compliance
The European Union's (EU) General Product Safety Regulation (GPSR) is a set
of rules that requires consumer products to be safe and our obligations to
ensure this.

If you have any concerns about our products, you can contact us on

ProductSafety@springernature.com

In case Publisher is established outside the EU, the EU authorized
representative is:

Springer Nature Customer Service Center GmbH
Europaplatz 3
69115 Heidelberg, Germany

www.ingramcontent.com/pod-product-compliance
Ingram Content Group UK Ltd.
Pitfield, Milton Keynes, MK11 3LW, UK
UKHW020756080726
473059UK00006B/1900